GLUTTONY WITHOUT GUILT

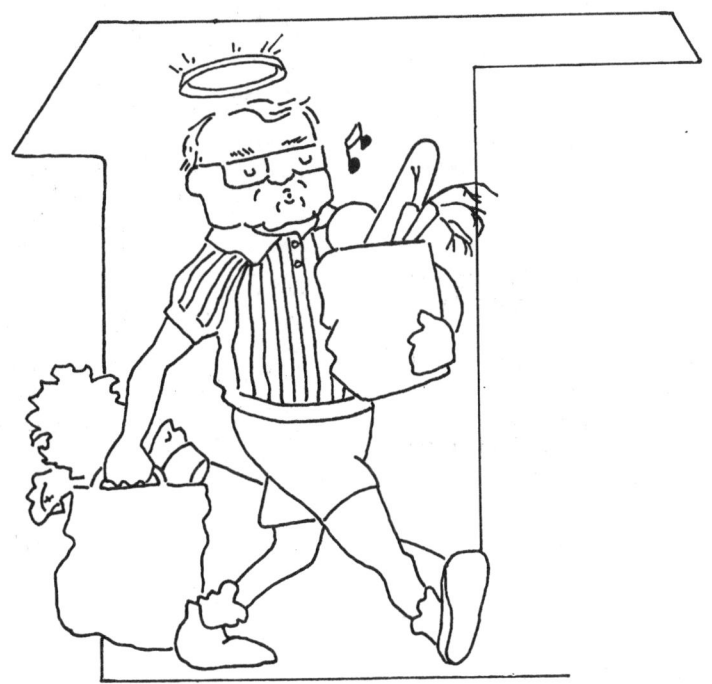

A Common-Sense Cookbook

By John Owen

Illustrated by Alice Owen

Cookbooks by John Owen

Intermediate Eater

Second Intermediate Eater

Gourmand Gutbusters

The Great Grub Hunt

The Seattle Cookbook
First Printing 1983
Second Printing 1985
Third Printing 1993 (Revised)
Fourth Printing 1994
Fifth Printing 1995

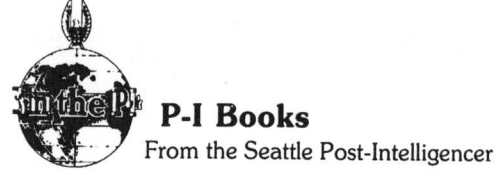

P-I Books
From the Seattle Post-Intelligencer

ISBN 0-9624559-6-2

TABLE OF CONTENTS

Bread and Breakfast 7

Soup 11

Salads 17

Vegetables 21

Casseroles 27

Beans and Rice 33

Appetizers 37

Italian Pasta and Asian Noodles 41

Poultry 45

Beef and Pork 55

Seafood 61

Shellfish 67

Desserts 73

OK, maybe you don't consider yourself a glutton . . .

But you like to eat, right? And if you are a typical American your body mass index (as computed by government scientists) approximates that of a 1957 Volkswagen bug.

Again, if you are a typical eager eater, you have also determined that the solution does not lie in diet plans which preach a caloric quotient based on the body temperature of a raw parsnip slice, divided by the number of radishes that have been placed upon your plate.

Your stomach knows when you introduce pretend food into the daily fare. Better you should fill the complaining organ with mashed pototoes. And the potatoes go down a lot easier with some chicken gravy. What you need to learn is this:

A LITTLE CHICKEN GRAVY DOESN'T MAKE YOU A BAD PERSON!

Honest. But what you should do is to mash the potatoes with some warmed skim milk and add seasoning to taste. Then create a no-fat gravy by mixing two tablespoons of Wondra Flour with a quarter cup of water. When smooth mix in a cup of chicken bouillon. Bring to a boil to thicken, then stir in some dried sage and maybe a squirt of Kitchen Bouquet.

Heat some turkey breast, plunk it on slices of bread next to the mashed potatoes, top with the gravy and you have a pretty darn good hot turkey sandwich. And you are still a good person.

"NUTS" AND BOLTS OF SENSIBLE NUTRITION

That kind of logic is incorporated into this cookbook in an attempt to simplify some diet rules that seem to confound even those food scientists who write them.

For example, one medical journal reports that the intake of nuts should be restricted because of the high oil content. Then another reports on a survey of elderly men, indicating that those who ate the most nuts lived longest.

Things like eggs and liver are bad for you, we've been told. Well, not as bad as we first thought, later studies have shown. The direct intake of cholesterol apparently is not as damaging as the consumption of saturated fats, which create cholesterol. Got it?

Maybe you have, maybe you haven't. Eliminating butter from your diet seems like a giant stride in the right direction so you substitute one of those new, healthy margarine brands on the market. Except that scientists have now discovered that trans-fatty acids, created when vegetable oils are converted into spreads, are really, really, REALLY bad for you. Maybe the butler (or the butter) didn't do it after all.

A little creative cooking, based on as much scientific research as a hungry person's mind can absorb, has resulted in these culinary tips which might help you avoid depression and malnutrition.

A NEW WAY TO APPEASE YOUR LUSTS

- If you live in the Northwest, you've already won the lottery. Because salmon may be the almost perfect protein because of the beneficial Omega 3 fatty acids the fish contains. If you wish to follow a low-fat diet you can also load up on pasta, beans, rice, soup, veggie stir-fries and other seafoods. There are chapters in this book devoted to each.

- Favor poultry (preferably skinned) or seafood over beef, lamb or pork. The number of recipes for each in this book reflect our preference.

- Limit your intake of butter and margarine. Between the two, butter may be preferable to margarine from a health standpoint. Where possible substitute olive or Canola oil in your cooking. If you think a dish desperately needs a buttery flavor, stir in a product known as Butter Buds before serving. If you still think the dish needs some butter, use some. Some desserts need it. Besides, you're a grown person and are allowed to choose. In fact the "b" word will be found in some of the recipe ingredients within this book. Just be aware of the options.

- Learn to read and interpret both the ingredients and the nutrition facts on the side of the package. Partially hydrogenated additives (in margarine, and in packaged items like potato chips, cookies and crackers) provide a warning signal. So do high levels of saturated fats. Pretend you are on an Easter egg roll or a mushroom hunt. You get bonus points if you discover a low-fat product that also tastes good.

- Shop for low-fat cheeses. To appease an uncontrollable cheese lust try melting slices of Healthy Choice American cheese in toasted cheese sandwiches. Velveeta also has a low-fat American cheese that is OK for these purposes.

- Substitute non-fat cream cheese and sour cream whenever possible. In most recipes you'll discover the taste and texture is virtually the same as the high-fat product.

- If you want to reduce your consumption of whole eggs substitute Second Nature in cooked dishes. Again, you probably won't notice the difference. This product is also eminently satisfactory for making French toast on a Sunday morning. (Add a little vanilla or almond extract to the egg mixture and dunk your bread in that.)

- For that same Sunday breakfast try Jimmy Dean's low-fat sausage. It contains hardly any grease but tastes just fine. Even better, create your own sausage "brand" using ground turkey breast. (I prefer the Turkey Store product with seven percent fat.) To lower the percentage even more I add dried bread crumbs, some Second Nature egg substitute and seasonings like salt, black pepper, sage and cayenne to achieve the right taste and texture for my homemade sausage.

- There are several recipes in this book for entrees using ground turkey breast. Before you buy it at the market, however, check the fat content. Turkey fat and skin might be included in the grind of some cheap brands.

- Try substituting "low-fat" mayo. You probably won't like the "fat-free" dressing. Matter of fact, I don't like it, either.

- If you need something besides jam on your morning toast try Promise Ultra margarine. It contains no fat, no trans fatty acids. You can't cook with it, but on toast, or melted into baked or mashed potatoes, it's not too bad.

- You'd be surprised at the improved taste and texture of some of the new brands of no-fat or low-fat ice cream or frozen yogurt products. Try them. You might like 'em.
- Try substituting low-fat canned milk for cream in soups or chowders. There is even a recipe for "cream" created out of skim milk and tofu in this book. I've used it in both soups and desserts. And although I thought I was a confirmed tofu skeptic, I really liked it.

So read the recipes, follow the directions as written or make the substitutes that are suggested here or which have been added to the list of ingredients, as a footnote.

There is occasional mention of brands I have used and enjoyed. The Intermediate Eater has no affiliation with any of the companies involved. I receive no free products. Jimmy Dean doesn't even send me a singing Christmas card.

*We're just trying to make shopping
(and enjoyable dieting)
a little easier for readers who ascribe to be
Gluttons Without Guilt.*

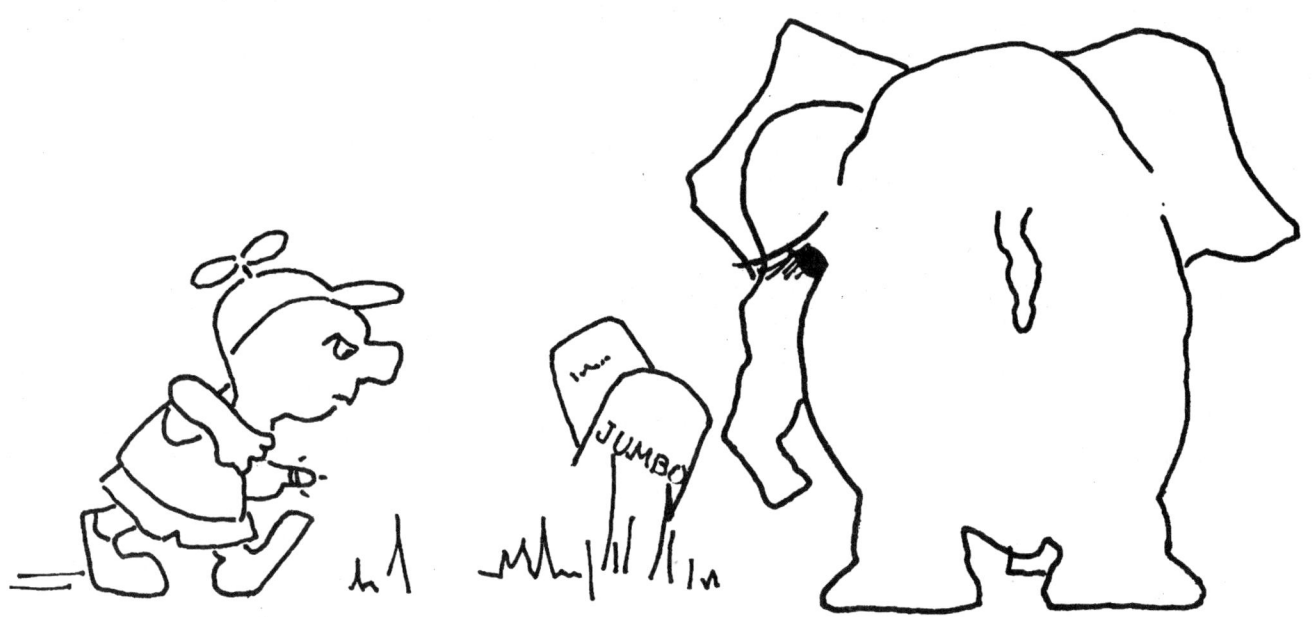

BREAD AND BREAKFAST

The Intermediate Eater harbors no personal grudge against the breakfast cereal manufacturers of America. What I harbor is more of a class-action grudge.

Cold breakfast cereal has never tasted good. There has never been any question about that among epicures and intellectuals. Granted, I ate some when I was a kid. But I had a reason. There was absolutely no other way I could come into the possession of an authentic Jack Armstrong pedometer, an instrument which allowed me to measure the exact distance between my home in Billings, Mont., and The Elephants Graveyard somewhere in darkest Africa.

OK, I never actually had occasion to walk from Billings to the Elephants Graveyard. But I was equipped for the trip, since I was also in possession of a Tom Mix Signal Arrowhead, which embodied a genuine working compass, magnifying and/or signal glass and a breath-operated emergency siren.

Do you know what I'm offered today, on the cereal boxes Alice the Artist persists in hauling home from the market? I'm offered 100 percent the recommended daily amount of Folate. I'm not even sure I want 0.4 mg a day of Folate, although the cereal box claims I should, especially if I'm "thinking about getting pregnant."

During the Age of Enlightenment, cereal box tops offered the choice of a Buck Rogers glow-in-the dark Venusian ring or a Captain Midnight Code-O-Graph.

Fat kids with no aspirations on Venus could at least send away for a Little Orphan Annie Ovaltine Shakeup Mug.

What are we offered today? Folate. And Fiber.

So I don't eat breakfast cereal any more. At least I don't eat it in its primitive form – cold and soggy from a 60-second soaking in skim milk.

If Alice insists we need a Folate and Fiber fix, I might mix up a batch of Capt. Midnight muffins. They contain ingredients from three cereal boxes, which in The Olden Days would have been good for a magic ring, a code pin and a pocket flashlight capable of summoning Major Steele's Amphibian Rescue Craft in moments of extreme danger.

Capt. Midnight Muffins

- 2 cups oatmeal
- 2 cups crumbled Shredded Wheat
- 2 cups All Bran
- 1 cup boiling water
- 1 cup canola oil
- 1 pound brown sugar
- 4 cups low-fat buttermilk
- 4 eggs, beaten
- 5 cups flour
- 5 teaspoons soda
- 1 teaspoon salt (or less)

Dump the oats, wheat and bran into a large bowl. Pour the boiling water over all, then add the oil, sugar and buttermilk.

Add the eggs (and, yes, you can use a substitute like Second Nature for all or part of your eggs.)

Dump in the flour, soda and salt and mix well.

Fill oiled muffin tins slightly more than half full and bake in a preheated 400-degree oven about 20 minutes, or until a toothpick comes out clean.

Cover the leftover batter and refrigerate. It will keep for almost a month and should furnish you with about four dozen muffins.

Bird-Feeder Muffins

- 8 ounces unprocessed bran
- 2½ cups flour
- 2½ teaspoons baking soda
- 1 teaspoon salt
- ½ teaspoon nutmeg
- ½ teaspoon allspice
- ½ teaspoon cinnamon
- 1 cup orange marmalade
- 1 cup honey
- 2 eggs, beaten
- 1 tablespoon vanilla
- ½ cup margarine, melted
- 1 pint buttermilk
- 2 cups raisins
- 2 apples, peeled, cored and chopped

Mix together dry ingredients. Dump in liquids and moosh until combined. Stir in fruit. Fill muffin cups (greased or containing muffin papers) 2/3 full and bake in 375-degree oven for 15 to 20 minutes.

Makes about three dozen muffins. The uncooked batter will keep in the refrigerator for a couple of weeks.

Great Western Muffins

- 7 cups bran flake cereal with raisins
- 3 cups sugar
- 5 cups flour
- 5 teaspoons baking soda
- 2 teaspoons salt
- 4 well-beaten eggs
- 1 cup cooking oil
- 1 quart buttermilk

In your largest bowl, mix together the cereal, sugar, flour, soda and salt. Add the eggs, oil and buttermilk. (I have used egg substitute and 1 percent buttermilk with good success.) Moosh all this around until blended. Then cover well and let it sit in the refrigerator until you arise the next morning. What you do then is to grease a muffin tin and fill each cup half full. Then shove into a preheated 375-degree oven for about 22 minutes, testing with that toothpick all cowboys keep in their vest pocket. As long as you keep the batter covered and refrigerated, it should provide about 48 muffins and a whole lot of breakfasts.

Route 101 Zucchini Bread

- 3 eggs
- 1 cup canola oil
- 1 cup white sugar
- 1 cup brown sugar, firmly packed
- 3 teaspoons maple flavoring
- 2 cups coarsely shredded zucchini
- 2½ cups flour, unsifted
- ½ cup toasted wheat germ
- 2 teaspoons baking soda
- 2 teaspoons salt
- ½ teaspoon baking powder
- 1 cup finely chopped walnuts
- 1/3 cup sesame seeds

Beat the eggs with a rotary mixer. Add the oil, sugars and maple flavoring, continuing to beat until thick and foamy. Stir in the zucchini with a back-scratcher from the Forest of Fudge souvenir shop. Mix together the flour, wheat germ, soda, salt, baking powder and walnuts. Stir into the zucchini mess just until blended.

Divide the batter between two greased and flour-dusted 5-inch-by-9-inch loaf pans. Sprinkle the sesame seeds over the tops. Bake in a pre-heated 350-degree oven for an hour, or until the bread passes the old toothpick test. Cool in pans 10 minutes, turn out onto wire racks and cool before serving.

Hawaiian Cornbread

- ¾ cup canola oil
- ¾ cup sugar
- 3 eggs
- ¼ teaspoon nutmeg
- 3 cups Bisquick
- 1 cup milk
- ¼ cup cornmeal
- 1 teaspoon vanilla

Cream together the oil, sugar, eggs and nutmeg. Stir in the Bisquick, milk, cornmeal and vanilla and mix thoroughly. Dump this muck into a greased, 9-inch by 12-inch baking pan and shove into a 325-degree oven for about 45 minutes, or until the bread pulls away from the sides of the pan. Let cool 10 minutes then cut in squares and serve with soup.

This is supposed to be the same cornbread featured at Stewart's Pharmacy, a landmark establishment in Waikiki up until the 1960s. In the authentic recipe, ½ cup of melted butter was poured over the top of the bread as soon as it was removed from the oven. I skipped the extra butter and it was still great cornbread.

Pumpkin Spread

- 1 pound can of pumpkin
- 1 teaspoon lemon juice
- 1 teaspoon lemon rind
- ½ cup orange juice
- ¾ cup brown sugar
- ⅛ teaspoon ground cloves
- ⅛ teaspoon ground ginger
- ⅛ teaspoon ground cinnamon
- Pinch of salt

Combine all the ingredients in a pot over high heat. When the ingredients begin to belch heavily, reduce the heat to low and simmer 30 minutes.

It's great spooned warm over baked squash. Refrigerate the rest and use as a topping for toast, muffins or zucchini bread.

In case you didn't know, pumpkin is loaded with beta carotene even when canned. It also contains iron, calcium and magnesium, and I wouldn't be surprised if it also removes fungus from your big toe.

Graham Bread

- 2 cups graham flour
- 1 cup whole wheat flour
- ½ cup sugar
- 1 teaspoon salt
- 2 teaspoon baking soda
- 2 cups buttermilk

Preheat oven to 400 degrees. Sift together dry ingredients. Add buttermilk and mix thoroughly. Pour the batter into a greased loaf pan. Shove the pan into the oven, immediately turn the thermostat down to 350 degrees and let bake for one hour.

Airline Loaves

- 1 cup canola oil
- 2 eggs
- 3 cups sugar
- 5 cups flour
- 4 teaspoons baking soda
- 1 teaspoon cinnamon
- 1 teaspoon cloves
- 1 teaspoon salt
- 1 large can (No. 2 ½) pumpkin
- 2 cups raisins
- 2 cups chopped walnuts

Mix together the first nine ingredients. When thoroughly combined stir in raisins and nuts.

Spray 8-inch-by-4-inch loaf pans with oil. Divide the batter among the pans. Bake for about 60 minutes in a 350-degree oven.

Edmonds Toast

- 6 large eggs
- ¼ cup milk
- 4 tablespoons orange juice
- 2 tablespoons fruit syrup
- ¼ teaspoon ground cinnamon
- ⅛ teaspoon ground nutmeg
- 6 thick slices sourdough bread

Beat the eggs (or use an egg substitute) and add the next five ingredients. (I used maraschino cherry syrup but use any fruit syrup that happens to be hanging around your refrigerator.)

Thoroughly soak the halved bread slices on both sides in the above muck.

Then fry on a grill lightly coated with canola oil and serve with syrup.

Cedar St. Corn Cakes

   1 egg
   ½ cup buttermilk
   ½ teaspoon baking soda
   ¾ cup corn meal (yellow or blue)
   ¼ cup flour
   1 teaspoon sugar
   2 tablespoons canola oil
   1 teaspoon baking powder
   ¼ teaspoon salt

Beat the egg, buttermilk and soda. Then beat in the corn meal, flour, sugar, oil, baking powder and salt until you have a smooth batter. If it is too thick, add buttermilk until you get the consistency you prefer. This should be enough batter for 14 small corn cakes. Cook on a griddle and serve with maple syrup. Or you can make a special syrup by mixing two parts honey with one part maple syrup, heating slowly, then adding a teaspoon of cinnamon.

(If you don't have buttermilk, just add 1 ½ teaspoons vinegar to sweet milk and let sit a moment.)

Puget Potato Cakes

   2½ cups leftover mashed potatoes
   2 lightly beaten eggs
   2 teaspoons minced capers
   12 olives (black or green) chopped
      Italian bread crumbs
      Salt as needed

Mix spuds with the eggs (or egg substitute), capers, olives and salt to taste. Form into cakes.

Coat both sides in the crumbs and fry in canola or olive oil about 4 minutes, turning once. Serves 4, maybe with some fried ham on the side.

Hash-brown Quiche

    Shredded potatoes
   1 cup ham, in cubes
   1 cup Swiss cheese, grated
   1 cup hot pepper cheese, grated
   2 eggs
   ½ cup half and half
   ¼ teaspoon seasoned salt

I've used this recipe with egg substitute and low-fat ham and it worked fine.

You can peel and grate your own potatoes or buy them at the market, frozen or in fresh pouches. You need enough to form the crust in a greased, 10-inch pie plate. Press the grated spuds in with your hands, brush with oil and then cook the potato crust for 25 minutes in a 425-degree oven.

Next you distribute the ham in the crust and scatter over the top the two cheeses. Beat the eggs with the half and half and seasoned salt and pour this mess over the pie.

Bake in a 350-degree oven for 30 to 40 minutes and let cool 5 minutes before you serve to three or four guests. This reheats pretty well. And if you want to turn the heat up, use two cups of pepper cheese and no Swiss.

Vitamin C Sources

- Grapefruit
- Oranges
- Strawberries
- Raspberries
- Tomatoes
- Hot red peppers
- Cantaloupe
- Broccoli

How Much Salt Is Too Much Salt?

You figure it out. I can't.

Salt (or sodium) has been linked to strokes, high blood pressure and hypertension. However, scientists admit they have not yet seen a study proving that a low-salt diet led to a drop in heart disease or stroke for any group that had been tracked.

Moreover, a four-year Cornell University study of 1,900 men with high blood pressure showed that those who had been using more than 10 grams of salt a day (the national average) had only one-fourth as many heart attacks as those who limited their salt to five grams or less.

Confused? Maybe you've been using too much pepper.

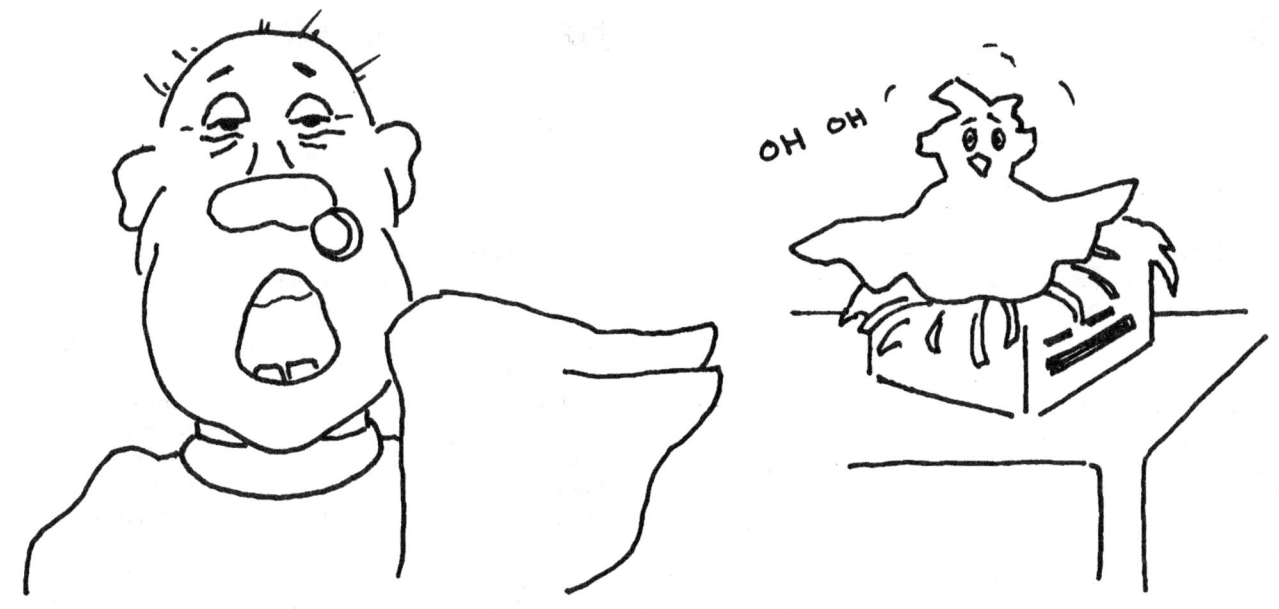

SOUP

I'm surprised nobody took the time to explain this to me before. I could have avoided a lot of awkward pauses on those occasions when I encountered somebody who looked, sounded and acted perfectly normal, but had a metal ring dangling from the nose.

You have to admit that it begs comment. But what do you say, "Nice nose ring?" They'd know it was a lie. If I really thought it was nice, I'd have one, too. And, as friends and acquaintances have noticed, I don't.

That may prove to be my problem. Only recently did I discover a likely and logical explanation for nose rings. I was enlightened by an article in *Health Magazine*.

The subject was the common cold. It seems the latest medical evidence suggests you can reduce or avoid illness if you will only remember to keep your hands away from your nose.

Kissing isn't liable to give you a cold, unless you sniff at the same time and why in the world would you do that? Colds are caused when rhinovirus lodges high up in your nasopharynx. And it is usually directed in that area by the hand.

So wash your hands during the cold season. And keep them away from you-know-where.

The problem is we forget and absent-mindedly rub, scratch or probe forbidden recesses.

Aha! But there is obviously a way to remember. Wear a ring in your nose, the bigger the better. In fact, a miniature copy of Big Ben might be appropriate during cold season. A warning gong would sound when you approached the forbidden area with a wandering hand.

For those of us who can't or (more accurately) won't wear rings, hope is faint. Yet we can reduce the length and severity of the common cold by eating, and inhaling, lots of chicken soup. Jewish mothers always knew best, after all. Scientists add that chicken soup containing garlic or strong spices might help even more, in relieving cold symptoms.

My contributions to medical science will be found on the following pages, without benefit of nose ring.

Chili Chicken Soup

  2½ pounds chicken pieces
  2   onions
      Celery tops
  1   tablespoon chili powder
  1   teaspoon Italian herbs
  2   teaspoons ground cumin
  3   minced cloves garlic
      Cayenne pepper to taste
  5   stalks celery, sliced
  5   carrots, sliced
  2   green bell peppers, seeded and cut
      in one-inch cubes
  1   cup dry noodles
  1   bunch cilantro (leaves only)
      Salt
      Chicken bouillon powder

I used chicken hind-quarter sections that were on special. You could use chicken thighs in the same amount. Cover with water. Quarter an onion and toss in some celery tops, too. Bring to a boil, let simmer 5 minutes, then cover, turn off heat and let the chicken sit in the water for at least an hour. When cool remove the chicken pieces, discard the skin, bones, the onion and celery tops. Return the meat to the broth, refrigerate overnight, then skim off and discard the layer of chicken fat.

When ready to cook, pour a cup of the chicken broth into a soup pot. Add the chili powder, Italian seasonings, cumin and garlic. Boil 1 minute, then add the rest of the reserved stock. You should have about 8 cups total. Add water if needed.

Simmer the carrots, celery and one chopped onion in the broth for 20 minutes. While this is happening, cook the noodles in salted water.

Add the green pepper to the other veggies in the pot and simmer another 10 minutes.

Taste the broth and add chicken bouillon powder and/or salt to taste. You can also add the cayenne at this point or, if your guests are exploding sneezes at varying velocities, let them add the red pepper themselves, after you have dished the soup into bowls.

Before you dish it up, add the cooked chicken pieces, the chopped cilantro leaves and the cooked and drained noodles to the pot and bring broth back to a simmer.

This will make about 10 bowls of "Jewish penicillin," which can be served with crusty French bread or warmed tortillas. Better yet, if it is the holiday season, you might want to Deck the Soup With Matzo Balls.

Onion Soup

Reconstitute two envelopes of onion soup, according to directions on the package. Add a cup of red wine, a bay leaf, a half teaspoon of sage and simmer for 20 minutes. If you want it thicker, whisk in a few puffs of Wondra flour.

Icicle Creek Soup

  5   cups white beans
  1   pound low-fat turkey ham, diced
  2   tablespoons canola oil
  1   large onion, chopped
  2   cups dry white wine
  2   cups plum tomatoes
  2½ quarts chicken stock
  3   cloves garlic, minced
  3   bay leaves
  2   teaspoons thyme
  2   teaspoons rosemary
      Salt, pepper

Soak the beans overnight and drain. Cover bottom of a large pot with oil and brown the ham. Remove meat and in the same pot saute the onion 3 minutes. Add the other ingredients plus the drained beans and simmer 2 hours.

Puree half the mixture and return to the pot. Simmer another 30 minutes.

Add the ham and salt and pepper to taste. This should provide a week's worth of soup, or about 15 servings.

Meat Ball Soup

  1   pound extra lean ground beef
  1   cup soft bread crumbs
  ¼   cup minced onion
  ¼   cup milk
  1   teaspoon salt
  1   teaspoon Worcestershire sauce
  1   egg, beaten
  2   cups water
  1½ cups sliced carrots
  1½ cups sliced onions
  2   tablespoons butter
  2   cans (10 ½ ounces each) condensed
      cream of potato soup
  1   teaspoon dill weed

Moosh together the ground beef, crumbs, minced onion, milk, one teaspoon of salt, Worcestershire and egg. Mix well and shape into small meatballs.

In a pot combine the potato soup, the water, carrots, onions and butter. Cover and simmer until veggies are tender, about 15 minutes. Add the meatballs, plopping them into the pot one by one. Cover pot and simmer another 20 minutes. Add salt to taste.

Serves four to six as a main dish, with a loaf of chewy bread. Sprinkle dill weed over soup.

Mustard Pea Soup

- 2 medium onions, chopped
- 5 carrots, diced
- 5 stalks celery, diced
- 1 pound split peas
- 4 quarts chicken stock
- ½ teaspoon Italian herbs
- 4 tablespoons flour
- ½ pound low-fat ham, diced
- 2 12-ounce cans low-fat evaporated milk
- 3 tablespoons prepared mustard
- Canola oil
- Salt, pepper to taste

Saute the onions, carrots and celery in about 3 tablespoons canola oil for about 10 minutes. Pour in the stock and add the split peas and herbs. Bring to a boil, then reduce heat, cover and cook about 90 minutes, stirring occasionally.

Heat 4 tablespoons oil in a saucepan and stir in the flour. Stir cook for about 3 minutes, then add some of the hot soup, stir until smooth, then return this mess to the pot, stirring to eliminate any remaining lumps as the soup thickens.

Add the ham, the evaporated milk and the mustard of your choice. You probably won't need to add any salt to this soup, but you can stir more mustard into your individual bowl. This should make 10 bowls of soup.

Welsh Soup

- 2 tablespoons butter (or canola oil)
- 2 green onions, chopped
- 3 cloves garlic, minced
- ¼ teaspoon dried thyme
- 3 leeks
- 3 carrots
- 2 turnips
- 2 stalks celery
- 8 cups chicken broth
- ½ pound new potatoes
- salt, pepper to taste
- Croutons

Heat the oil or butter in a soup pot and saute the green onions, garlic and thyme a couple of minutes, making sure the garlic doesn't burn.

Add to the pot the white and light-green parts of the leeks (chopped) and both the carrots and turnips, which have first been peeled and diced. Toss in the diced celery, too. Saute this mess about 5 minutes, then add the chicken stock and the potatoes, diced.

You can then simmer this soup from 20 minutes to an hour. Sprinkle with parsley and add salt and pepper to taste.

This will serve four as a main dish, more as a first course, with the croutons sprinkled over the top.

Portuguese Bean Soup

- 1½ cups dry white beans
- 1 cup diced ham
- ½ teaspoon allspice
- 1 large onion, chopped
- 2 large carrots, sliced
- 1 large can (1 pound, 12 ounces) crushed tomatoes
- 1 can tomato soup
- 2 to 3 potatoes, peeled and cubed
- ½ a green cabbage, cut in cubes
- 1 teaspoon Worcestershire sauce
- 2 chicken bouillon cubes
- ⅓ cup chopped tops of green onions
- 1 10-ounce hunk of Portuguese sausage

Soak the beans overnight. Next day drain off the water and put the beans in a pot with 5 cups of fresh water. Bring to a boil, then pour this water off, too, and re-cover the beans with 5 cups fresh water plus the ham, allspice and onion. Cook until the beans are almost (but not quite) tender. Add the tomatoes, soup, carrots, potatoes, cabbage, green onion tops, the Worcestershire sauce, bouillon cubes and the sausage, in ¼-inch slices.

Simmer until the vegetables and beans are done. Add salt and pepper to taste.

Portuguese sausage, or linguica, has a slightly sweet flavor. You can often find it frozen at Asian grocery stores or markets. But I have used Healthy Choice low-fat smoked sausage and I don't think the soup suffered at all. This soup should provide six main-course servings or 10 cups to start a meal.

If you want to simplify this dish eliminate the dry beans and cook all the other ingredients until tender, adding drained kidney beans (1 or 2 cans) at the end.

Quick Veggie Soup

- 5 carrots, chopped
- 3 stalks celery, chopped
- 1 medium onion, chopped
- 1 package (10 ounces) frozen corn
- 6 ounces frozen green beans
- 4 cups chicken broth
- 1 can (14 ounces) undrained tomatoes, busted up
- ½ teaspoon Italian herbs
- 1 can (15 ounces) barbecue-style beans
- Salt, pepper to taste

Dump the first eight ingredients in a soup pot, bring to a boil and simmer about 30 minutes, or until carrots are tender. Add the beans with sauce. I prefer S&W's Texas-style BBQ beans to add some zest to the stock. Add salt and pepper to taste.

Punjabi Soup

     2 cups mixed dried beans
    12 cups chicken broth
     2 onions, chopped
     2 cups celery, chopped
     2 cups carrots, sliced
     4 teaspoons curry powder
     2 teaspoons ground turmeric
       Salt, pepper
    ¼ pound ham, cut in small cubes

Cover the beans with an inch of water. Bring to a boil for two minutes, then turn off the heat and let the beans sit, covered, for an hour.

Drain the beans and add 10 cups of chicken broth, vegetables, curry and turmeric. Bring to a simmer on stove for about 45 minutes or until beans are just tender.

Puree three-quarters of the beans in a blender or processor and return to the pot. Add salt and pepper to taste, plus the ham cubes. Reheat and this will make eight to 10 bowls of soup. If the soup is too thick, add all or part of the remaining two cups of chicken broth.

2000 Year Soup

     8 cloves garlic, peeled
     6 cups clam nectar
     2 medium potatoes
     1 cup chopped canned tomatoes
     1 pound bay scallops
    ¾ cup tofu
     1 cup skim milk
       Salt if needed
       Cayenne pepper

Try to find quart-sized cans of clam juice in a food specialty shop unless you have been steaming your own clams and saving the nectar in your freezer.

OK, what you do is to pour two cups of nectar into your soup pot along with the garlic and the drained tomatoes (with most of the seeds spooned off).

Bring to a boil, reduce heat and simmer 10 minutes.

Peel and cut the potatoes into small cubes and toss into the pot, too. When they are soft (about 15 minutes) pour this whole mess into a blender and process until smooth.

Pour back into the pot and in the same blender or processor plunk the tofu and skim milk. Process for a full minute. Then stir this into the soup and add remaining clam nectar. When mixture is hot again add the scallops. When they are done (about four minutes) add salt if needed then spoon this up into bowls (four to six) and allow guests to sprinkle a little cayenne over the top if they desire. With biscuits, a salad and dessert this is a complete meal.

Yakima Valley Chili

     1 pound small red beans
     2 tablespoons oil
     2 large onions, chopped
     4 cloves garlic, minced
     2 large green peppers, chopped
     2 medium carrots, peeled and chopped
    35 ounces chopped tomatoes with can juices
     1 cup tomato sauce
     3 tablespoons chili powder
     1 tablespoon ground cumin
     1 teaspoon oregano
    ⅛ teaspoon cayenne, or to taste
     2 chicken bouillon cubes

Pour boiling water over the beans and let sit an hour. Drain, cover with new water and partially cook the beans 45 minutes. Drain and set aside.

Heat oil in your chili pot. Add the onions, garlic, carrots and green peppers. If you like extra-hot chili, add one or two seeded and minced jalapeno peppers at this point.

Reduce heat and cook until the veggies have softened. Add the drained beans, two cups of water, the tomatoes, tomato sauce, bouillon and spices. Simmer 90 minutes. Add salt to taste.

If you like your chili thinner than this, add some water. If you want it thicker, slowly stir in Wondra flour until it's just right.

If you like ground beef in your chili, brown it in the pot just before you add the onions, garlic, carrots and peppers.

Lucky's Tomato Soup

     1 can Campbell's
    ½ teaspoon garlic powder
     1 tablespoon parsley, chopped
     2 pinches of oregano
       dash of curry powder
       another dash of chili powder
       a pinch of poultry seasoning

Got that? To the soup (diluted with a can of water) you are adding three pinches, two dashes, a dab of this and a bit of that. Heat and (guess what?) You've got tomato soup with character.

Garbure

    3   tablespoons olive oil
    3   carrots, sliced
    3   leaks (white part only) cut in quarter-inch slices
    2   cups chopped cabbage
    2   stalks celery, sliced
    1   teaspoon salt
    ½   teaspoon sugar
    7   cups water
    5   teaspoons beef bouillon powder
    2   cups cooked white beans
    2   potatoes, peeled and cubed
    ½   cup frozen green peas
        Buttered French bread
        Swiss cheese, grated

Heat the olive oil in a soup pot. Dump in the carrots, leeks, cabbage, celery, salt and sugar. Cover and cook over low heat 30 minutes.

Add to the pot the water and bouillon powder.

Bring the liquid to a boil and add the potatoes. Cover and simmer 45 minutes.

Remove half the vegetables from the pot and dump into a blender. Add half the cooked white beans. Puree with as much pot broth as needed, then return this sludge to the pot. Add the rest of the white beans and the frozen peas.

Let everything heat up again for about five minutes. Add freshly ground black pepper and, if you wish, some more salt or garlic salt to taste.

This will make about six bowls. For each guest, fry on both sides the buttered French bread and float one in each bowl. Top with grated Swiss cheese.

Put all the bowls on a cookie sheet and shove under an oven broiler until the cheese melts.

Curried Lentil Soup

    1   cup lentils
    1   onion, minced
    2   garlic cloves, minced
    2   carrots, peeled and diced
    1   stalk celery, diced
    10 cups chicken broth
    1   tablespoon curry powder
    1   large potato, peeled and diced
    1   bunch spinach, stemmed and chopped
    1   tablespoon red wine vinegar
        Plain yogurt

Wash the lentils a couple of times, then dump them into a soup pot with the onion, garlic, carrots, celery, curry powder and 6 cups of broth. Bring to a boil, reduce heat and simmer partially covered for 2 hours.

Add the potato, spinach and the rest of the stock and simmer another 2 hours uncovered. Add vinegar, salt to your taste and add more broth if you think it needs some.

Serve with a dollop of yogurt in each bowl.

Pea and Barley Bowl

    1½ cups split peas
    1   small onion, chopped
    1   large carrot, diced
    1   rib celery, diced
    1   clove garlic, minced
    7   cups chicken broth
    ½   cup barley
        Salt, pepper to taste

Combine in a pot the split peas, onion, carrot, celery, garlic and 6 cups broth. Bring to a boil and simmer uncovered for an hour, stirring once or twice and adding water to thin as needed.

Meanwhile, in a saucepan cook the barley in 1 cup broth 40-60 minutes or until tender.

Puree the split pea glunk and mix with the barley, salt and pepper.

Filibuster Chili

    4   cups black beans
    2   tablespoons cumin seed
    1   tablespoon oregano
    1   teaspoon sage
    2   medium onions, chopped
    1   large green pepper, seeded and chopped
    2   cloves garlic, minced
    ¼   cup olive oil
    1   teaspoon cayenne pepper
    1   tablespoon paprika
    1   teaspoon salt
    3   cups canned tomatoes, smashed
    ⅓   cup bottled jalapeno slices, minced
        Grated cheddar cheese
        Chopped cilantro

Soak the beans overnight, discard and replace the water and cook the beans until tender. Drain, saving a cup of the pot water.

Dump the cumin, oregano and sage in a small cake pan and put in a 350-degree oven for 10 minutes.

Heat the oil, add the onions, green pepper, garlic and the toasted herbs.

When the onions have softened add the tomatoes, jalapenos, the cooked beans and the cup of pot liquid. Add the salt, paprika and the cayenne, a quarter teaspoon at a time so you can decide exactly how hot you want the chili. I think a teaspoon is about right. It might also need more salt.

Simmer this mess for at least 30 minutes, adding liquid if you think it needs some. When it's ready to serve put some grated cheddar on the bottom of each bowl, spoon on the chili and top with chopped cilantro. You can also add sour cream and chopped onion, but then it no longer qualifies as either a chili or a soup. It's a salad.

Mulligaturkey Soup

- 1 turkey carcass
- 3 quarts water
- 3 teaspoons salt
- 3 teaspoons curry powder
- ½ teaspoon mace
- ½ teaspoon ground cloves
- 1 teaspoon pepper
- ½ cup chopped parsley
- 3 onions, chopped
- 3 carrots, sliced
- 3 stalks celery, sliced
- 2 green peppers, seeded and chopped
- 2 tart apples, pared and sliced
- ⅓ cup butter (or canola oil)
- 1 cup flour
- 1 24-ounce can tomatoes

Bust up the bones with a sockful of quarters until they – the bones, not the quarters – fit into the pot and are completely covered by the water. Add the salt, curry, mace, cloves and pepper. Cover and simmer 45 minutes.

Remove the turkey from the broth to cool. Discard the bones and skin and cut the meat into hunks.

In a saucepan heat the butter or oil, then cook the onion, carrot, celery, green pepper and apple until tender.

Stir in the flour, add a quart of the warm stock and stir until it has thickened. Return this glunk to the large soup pot with the remaining stock, add the tomatoes (which have been run once through the blender), the parsley and the turkey meat. Bring to a boil, reduce heat and simmer another hour.

Taste to see if it needs more salt and serve in large bowls.

Oyster Stew

- 3 tablespoons butter
- ½ teaspoon Worcestershire sauce
- ½ teaspoon celery salt
- 20 ounces of fresh oysters
- 24 ounces cream (or two cans lowfat evaporated milk)
- Salt, pepper
- Paprika

Heat the butter in a pot and add the Worcestershire and celery salt. Stir ingredients of pan, then dump in the oysters and cook just until they begin to firm up. (You can use small oysters or, for much less price, the medium oysters, cut into two or three pieces.)

Pour in the cream or evaporated milk and, when heated just below boiling, add salt and pepper to taste and dish up into two bowls. Scatter paprika over the top of each bowl and, if you wish, float a bit of butter on top.

Clam Chowder With Leeks

- cooking oil
- 3 large leeks, washed
- 1½ pounds red-skinned new potatoes
- ¼ cup flour
- 3 cups chicken broth
- 1 teaspoon thyme leaves
- Pepper, salt
- 3 cups (6 ounces each) chopped clams
- 3 cups cream, whole milk or low-fat canned, evaporated milk

Thinly slice the white and light green parts of the leeks, discarding the rest. Cut the unpeeled spuds into half-inch cubes.

In a soup pot, cook the leeks in a bit of olive or canola oil for four minutes. Sprinkle with flour and moosh it around in the pot. Stir in the broth, thyme and potatoes. Bring to a boil, lower heat and simmer until the spuds are tender. Add the milk or cream and the clams, including the nectar.

Heat, stirring, until steaming but not boiling. Taste to see if it needs salt and add a good grinding of pepper.

If you have prejudices against canned milk, sprinkle your portion with some mixture like Tony Chachere's Creole seasoning. In the oyster stew recipe, the Worcestershire sauce and celery salt serve the same function.

The clam chowder recipe should serve six.

Sweet Corn Soup

- 1 tablespoon canola oil
- 1 small onion, chopped
- 1 clove garlic, minced
- Corn scraped off six large, leftover cooked ears
- 5 cups chicken broth
- 2 teaspoons dried basil, or three tablespoons chopped fresh
- Pinch of sugar
- 1 slice of ham, chopped
- Tabasco sauce
- Fresh basil or cilantro

Heat the oil in your soup pot. Add the onion and garlic. Cook gently, covered, about 8 minutes.

Add corn, chicken broth, basil and sugar, raise heat and simmer, partially covered, 25 minutes.

Slop half of this mess into a food blender and, well, don't just stand there. Blend!

Return blender ingredients to soup pot. Add ham (not more than a quarter pound), reheat and serve, with Tabasco to taste and with fresh basil or cilantro scattered over the top of each bowl. Serves 4 as a main course, with hot bread and a salad.

SALADS

Read any good nutrition magazines lately? These publications have become more thought-provoking than the Sports Illustrated swimsuit issue.

"Wow, Great Metabolism!" a recent vitamin ad in one such journal is headlined over a photo of a bronzed lady in a revealing Spandex swimsuit stretched backward over a beach log. Boy, she looks healthy!

"Stimulate metabolism!" suggests yet another full-page ad in the same issue. It shows a young woman, in a red swimsuit, at the beach.

"Turn up your metabolism and turn a few heads," yet another vitamin pitch is headed. Dominating the page is the photo of a blonde, in a red swimsuit, at the beach.

The dictionary definition of metabolism deals with the buildup and destruction of protoplasm. Nothing at all about beach parties and red swimsuits.

Oh, yeah? (Wink wink.) Check out that metabolism!

Has this become just another buzz word to sell us products medical science isn't sure we really need?

Keep a firm grip on your wallet whenever you hear (or read) terms like "ancient healing," "nature's own" or "earth friendly." Each adjective or adverb adds $4.85 to the package price.

And consider the conflicting claims in such magazines suggesting that the healthiest people in the world come from India, Sweden, the Amazon rain forest, Navajo hogans or Chinese ginseng ranches.

What we do know is that garlic is a miracle drug, not in tiny capsules but mixed with things like lettuce, tomatoes and onion.

How do we know? I think I read it somewhere in a magazine.

There is also a surprise ending in the culinary mystery. Because we now have been told that there is one thing worse than high cholesterol. It's low cholesterol.

Don't give me that funny look.

If you disagree, direct your indignation at the people in the white coats.

Research funded by the French government linked very low cholesterol with depression. A Dutch research group agreed and reported those in the lowest one-third on the cholesterol scale were 2.4 times more likely to die from suicide, accidents or other violent events than those in the upper third.

I know one thing for sure. A steady diet of raw carrots and celery sticks would depress me. It might even prompt me to rob a meat market, certainly an invitation to violent death. Butchers aren't waving ostrich feathers over those haunches of beef.

Artichoke Salad

- ½ cup mayonnaise
- 1 tablespoon capers
- 1 clove garlic, minced
- 1 teaspoon curry powder
- ¼ teaspoon Worcestershire sauce
- 1 splat of Tabasco sauce
- ½ teaspoon dry mustard
- 1 jar (six ounces) marinated artichoke hearts, drained
- 2 quarts spinach leaves

Stir together the mayo (you can use a low-fat brand) with capers, garlic, curry, Worcestershire, Tabasco and mustard, refrigerate.

When you are ready to eat tear the spinach leaves into bite-sized pieces. Dice the artichoke and combine the two in a salad bowl. Add the dressing and toss. Serves four.

Chickadee Salad

- 2 cups bow-tie pasta
- 1½ cups frozen peas
- ½ cup mayonnaise
- 2 tablespoons Dijon mustard
- ¼ cup minced mint leaves
- ¼ cup minced green onions
- 2 tablespoons lemon juice
- 1 cup finely chopped celery
- 1 pound leftover salmon (or canned red salmon) in chunks

Cook pasta in salted water and cool. Mix the mayonnaise and Dijon, mint and lemon juice. Combine all the ingredients and serve chilled or at room temperature.

Picnic Potato Salad

- 3 pounds new red potatoes
- 1 small red onion
- 1 cup celery, diced
- 1 large, tart apple
- 18 pimento-stuffed green olives
- ⅓ cup chopped sweet pickle
- 1½ cups mayonnaise
- 1 teaspoon Dijon mustard
- 2 tablespoons white vinegar
- 1 teaspoon bottled steak sauce
- Salt, pepper if needed

Boil the spuds (which incidentally contain vitamins A, B-6 and potassium) until you can stick a fork in 'em. Drain and, if they are perfectly cooked, cool immediately in cold water.

Drain and chop the unpeeled potatoes when cool. Thinly slice the onion (calcium and iron.) Dice the celery (potassium and phosphorus) and the cored but unpeeled apple (hemicellulose and lignin). Slice the olives, including all the Vitamin A and iron.

OK, in a large serving dish or pot combine the potatoes, onion, celery, apple and pickle.

Moosh together in a small bowl the mayo, mustard, vinegar and steak sauce.

Mix into the potato mixture. Add salt and pepper if needed. Top with the sliced pimento olives.

Cover and refrigerate. It can be kept all day or over night. This will provide about 10 servings.

Company Chicken Salad

Salad:

- 1 pound boned and skinned chicken breasts
- ¼ cup olive oil
- 3 tablespoons lemon juice
- 1 clove garlic, minced
- 2 tablespoons dried oregano
- Salt, pepper
- ½ pound spinach fettuccine
- ½ pound feta cheese, crumbled
- 3 tomatoes, chopped
- ½ cup Greek olives
- ½ cup fresh parsley, chopped
- ¼ cup pine nuts, toasted

Marinade:

- ¼ cup olive oil
- 3 tablespoons lemon juice
- 1 clove garlic, minced
- 2 or 3 splats of Tabasco sauce
- 1 tablespoon dried oregano
- Salt, pepper

Moosh together the marinade ingredients and let the raw chicken sit in this swamp for an hour or two, refrigerated. Discard the marinade and grill the chicken until barely done, or bake 30 minutes in a 325-degree oven. Cool and cut into thin strips.

Cook the fettuccine until barely done, then plunge into cold water. Drain the pasta and pat dry with paper towels.

Dump the chicken and pasta into a bowl and add the tomatoes, feta cheese, olives and the other items in the top list of ingredients. Toss salad and serve at room temperature to 4 to 6 guests.

If any of your guests is on a chicken-free, pasta-free diet, give 'em a carrot to suck on while the rest of you do some serious eating.

A Greek Salad

    3 cups snow peas
    ½ cup cubed feta cheese
    4 teaspoons minced red onion
    1 teaspoon minced garlic
    1 tomato, diced
    4 tablespoons chopped walnuts
    4 tablespoons freshly grated Parmesan cheese

Combine all ingredients in a bowl.
Use as much of the following dressing as needed and save the rest for your next salad.

Dressing:

    ¼ cup fresh mint
    1 teaspoon minced garlic
    ¼ cup white wine vinegar
    Salt, pepper
    ½ cup olive oil

Combine mint, garlic, vinegar, salt and pepper in a processor. While running slowly, add the oil. Toss the salad and refrigerate until dinner time.

Coyote Salad

    3 cups cooked and shredded chicken breast meat
    ½ pound pea pods
    2 tablespoons sesame seeds
    ¼ cup canola oil
    3 tablespoons lemon juice
    2 tablespoons soy sauce
    2 tablespoons white wine vinegar
    3 cloves garlic, pressed
    1 tablespoon minced fresh ginger root
    1 cup celery, diced
    ⅓ cup fresh cilantro leaves
    2 green onions, including tops, diced
    1 tomato, cut in eighths

Remove the ends and strings from the pea pods, then throw into a pot of boiling water for 90 seconds. Drain the pods and plunge into cold water.

Toast the sesame seeds three minutes in a skillet over medium heat. Remove when they start to brown and toss seeds into a small bowl. Add the oil, lemon juice, soy sauce, vinegar, garlic and the ginger. In a large bowl, plunk the chicken, celery and cilantro. Mix in the dressing.

Spread the pea pods on four plates like the spokes on a wheel. Grab handfuls of the chicken gloop and plunk in the center of each plate. Scatter the green onions over the top and decorate the plates with the slices of tomato.

Potato-Pea Puget Salad

    1 pound frozen green peas, thawed
    5 large potatoes, cooked, peeled and cubed
    1 bunch green onions, chopped
    4 tablespoons wine vinegar
    1 clove garlic
    1 tablespoon fresh oregano (or ½ teaspoon dried)
    1 tablespoon fresh thyme (or ½ teaspoon dried)
    Salt, pepper
    ½ cup olive oil
    Tomato wedges
    1 small red onion, thinly sliced
    1 small green pepper, sliced into rings

Dump the spuds, peas and green onions into a bowl.

In a smaller bowl, moosh together the vinegar, garlic, herbs, salt and pepper. Beat in the olive oil. Pour this sludge over the vegetables, toss and chill.

Serve with the tomato wedges, sliced red onion and green pepper rings.

Charlie's Salad

    2 cans tuna
    12 ounces noodles or pasta of your choice
    1 cup grated carrot
    2 cups drained sauerkraut
    1 cup shredded cheddar cheese
    1 cup diced celery
    1 green pepper, seeded and chopped
    3 tablespoons grated onion
    ½ cup diced dill pickle
    mayonnaise

If you are a big spender you may use albacore tuna. And despite your misgivings your guests are NOT going to squirm and pout once they discover the sauerkraut. They won't even know what it is. They'll just know it's good.

Mix everything together, add mayo to moisten and this should make eight portions.

Mexican Shrimp Salad

1 red onion
1 green pepper
1 red pepper
3 fresh tomatoes
1 pound small shrimp
½ cup halved black olives
½ cup halved green olives
½ cup olive oil
⅓ cup lemon juice
1 minced clove garlic
2 tablespoons minced cilantro leaves
1 jalapeno pepper, minced
  salt, pepper

Cut the onion and peppers into julienne strips. Chop the tomatoes.
Mix all ingredients in a large bowl or extra-large sombrero. Mix and refrigerate several hours. This should provide six or more portions.

Gazpacho Guadalahara

2 large tomatoes
1 cucumber
1 onion
1 green pepper
2 cloves garlic, minced
3 cups tomato juice
¼ cup olive oil
⅓ cup red wine vinegar
¼ teaspoon Tabasco sauce
1½ teaspoons salt
⅛ teaspoon freshly ground black pepper
¼ cup chopped chives
1 cup garlic croutons

In a blender combine 1 large tomato, ½ of a cucumber ½ an onion, one-quarter of a green pepper, the garlic and a half cup of tomato juice. Blend at high speed 30 seconds. Pour into a large bowl and add another 2 ½ cups of tomato juice plus the olive oil, vinegar, Tabasco, salt and pepper. Refrigerate until well chilled.
Just before serving add 1 chopped tomato, half an onion chopped, half a cuke chopped, three-fourths of a green pepper chopped and sprinkle with chives and garlic croutons.

Rice-Cabbage Salad

2 tablespoons canola oil
2 cloves garlic, pureed
1 minced onion
2 cups quick brown rice
2½ cups beef broth
1 bay leaf
2 slices fresh ginger
1 teaspoon pepper
4 cups shredded cabbage
2 cups shredded carrots
½ cup fresh cilantro
¼ cup fresh mint leaves
½ cup lemon juice
½ cup more canola oil
2 teaspoons sugar

Pour the two tablespoons of oil into a pot. Add the rice, onion and garlic.
Stir-cook five minutes. Add the broth, bay leaf, ginger and pepper. Bring to a boil then cover and simmer about 15 minutes or until liquid is absorbed.
Remove and discard the bay leaf and ginger slices.
Dish rice into a serving plate. Let it, and the economy, cool off.
Make a dressing from the minced cilantro, the minced mint, the lemon juice, the half cup canola oil and sugar. Mix this with the cabbage and carrots. Mix the vegetables in with the rice, using two forks to blend. Serve at room temperature.

Jimica Salad

4 tablespoons white wine vinegar
½ teaspoon paprika
¼ teaspoon salt
¼ teaspoon pepper
4 tablespoons canola oil
1 clove garlic, minced
2 teaspoons sugar
1 small jicama, peeled and sliced
4 satsuma oranges, peeled and sectioned

Blend the first seven ingredients for the dressing. Toss with the satsumas and jicama and serve atop lettuce leaves.

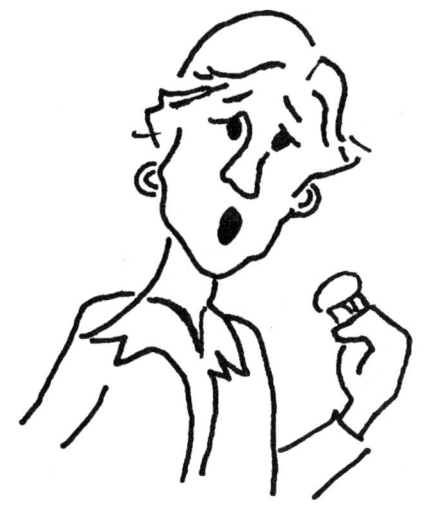
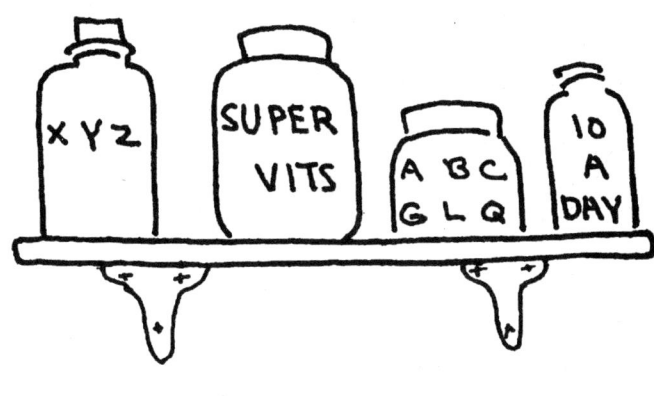

VEGETABLES

Alice the Artist reads and notes all the latest nutritional information.
 She has discovered so many different vitamins, letters of the alphabet have all been exhausted.
 For identification purposes, it soon will be necessary for her to assign license plates to her vitamin bottles, as in: B12-WOW (I'd rather be shopping at Nature's Pantry.)
 There is just one problem, relating to Alice's nutritional research: She can't swallow pills.
 I'm not talking about the golf ball-sized pills they give elephants to inhibit the formation of rust on their trunk locks. Alice can't swallow an aspirin without spewing water across the room, kicking furniture, scaring the cat and setting off the burglar alarm.
 The 911 operator stands on alert whenever she is informed by phone that Alice is holding a handful of vitamins.
 There should be an easier way. And there is. There is no valid reason why Alice cannot drink her vitamins, unless she chooses to bite or lick them.
 You see, there is a new nutritional slogan: "Broccoli each day keeps the doctors away."
 Broccoli contains vitamins A, C, B1, B2, B6, E plus niacin, calcium, iron, folic acid, phosphorus, magnesium, zinc, cooper and pantothenic acid.
 Oh, yeah, researchers at Johns Hopkins University School of Medicine recently isolated an ingredient in broccoli called sulforaphane, which works to stimulate the production of anti-cancer enzymes.
 Possibly with Alice the Artist in mind, the chef at a Seattle restaurant recently created a menu featuring broccoli soup, broccoli pate, broccoli souffle, broccoli bread cheese rolls and broccoli sponge cake with broccoli butter cream. And to go with the cake, he created a batch of broccoli ice cream.
 Most cooks just grab a bunch of broccoli off a supermarket counter and then hold it under hot water until it has drowned. That's probably how broccoli got a bad reputation in the George Bush family.
 Personally, I prefer my sulforaphane stir-fried with fresh ginger in a recipe like the one you'll find on the next page.

Ginger Broccoli

- 1 head broccoli, separated into florets
- 2 tablespoons canola or olive oil
- 3 green onions, chopped, including green part
- 1 clove garlic, minced
- 1 tablespoon fresh ginger root, minced
- 2 tablespoons oyster sauce

Heat the oil in a skillet and stir-fry the green onions, garlic and ginger 1 minute. Add the broccoli and stir-fry until tender. Add the oyster sauce, stir and cook another minute and serve.

Multi-Vitamin Broccoli

- 3 tablespoons Dijon mustard
- juice of one lemon
- ½ teaspoon paprika
- ¼ teaspoon cayenne pepper
- 1 tablespoon olive oil
- salt
- three cups of broccoli florets

Combine mustard, lemon juice, paprika, cayenne and olive oil. Steam the broccoli over boiling water until barely tender. Dump into a bowl, toss with the sauce and add salt if needed. Serves 4 or more.

Eat-Your Broccoli

- 2 tablespoons canola oil
- ¾ pound broccoli
- 1¼ cups sliced mushrooms
- 1 large carrot
- 1 clove garlic, minced
- 1 teaspoon grated lemon rind
- ½ teaspoon salt
- ¼ teaspoon dried thyme

Cut the broccoli florets from the stalks, then cut the stalks into quarter-inch slices. Peel the carrot and cut into julienne strips.

Heat the oil in a skillet and add the broccoli stalks, the carrot, the garlic, lemon rind, salt and thyme. Cook two minutes then dump in the florets and the mushrooms and continue to saute for two or three more minutes. Serves 4.

Safari Stir-Fry

- 2 tablespoons sherry
- 1 tablespoon oyster sauce
- ¼ cup chicken broth
- 1 tablespoon soy sauce
- 6 ounces (or two cups) dry noodles
- 2 tablespoons canola oil
- 2 tablespoons minced green onions
- 1 teaspoon minced ginger root
- 1 teaspoon minced garlic
- 1 cup mushrooms, thickly sliced
- ½ of a sweet red pepper, thinly sliced
- 1 cup bean sprouts
- 2 cups bok choy (white and green parts) thinly sliced
- 1 cup pea pods
- 2 teaspoons cornstarch

Mix the first four ingredients.

Use whatever stir-fry noodles you prefer, like yaki soba. Or you can use thin spaghetti, broken in half. Cook in boiling salted water until barely done. Drain thoroughly.

Pour a bit of oil in a hot skillet or wok and toss in the cooked noodles.

Flip them once or twice but do not stir. When noodles begin to scorch, turn out onto a serving platter and shove into a warm oven.

Reduce heat under your skillet or pan, and add a bit more oil. Saute the green onions for 1 minute. Add the garlic and ginger and cook another 30 seconds. Increase heat and add the mushrooms, pepper slices, bean sprouts, bok choy and pea pods. Stir-fry for 1 minute.

Mix 2 teaspoons of cornstarch in with the soy-sherry mixture. Stir, then pour over the veggies. Stir-cook until the sauce thickens, then pour this mess over the noodles and this will serve two to three.

Carolina Collards

- 5 pounds greens
- 2 tablespoons olive oil
- 1 large onion, chopped
- 3 cloves garlic, minced
- 2 cups water
- ½ pound ham, shredded
- 2 tablespoons sugar
- Cayenne pepper

While whistling the Tar Heel fight song, thoroughly wash the collard greens to remove all that Carolina mud. Cut off and discard the largest stems. Then cut the greens into inch-wide strips.

Heat the oil in a large pot. Saute the onions and garlic for two minutes.

Stir in the water, ham and sugar and simmer three minutes. Add the greens, cover the pot and let it simmer over low heat for about an hour. (Add more water if needed.) Sprinkle the greens with cayenne pepper to taste and stir everything around again. This should serve six.

Twice Cooked Spuds

Baking potatoes
Canola oil
Salt, pepper

Cook the unpeeled spuds in water to cover for 25 minutes. Remove, drain and refrigerate.
Half an hour before dinner is ready, cut the spuds into 1/8-inch slices.
Lay out in lines on a greased cookie sheet, slightly overlapping. Brush with oil and sprinkle with salt and pepper.
Bake in a 375-degree oven for 25 minutes, or until golden.

Cheese Potatoes

6 cups mashed potatoes
2 cloves garlic, pureed
1 can cheese soup
2 teaspoons salt
1/3 cup milk
1½ cups bread crumbs
2 tablespoons butter

Dump the undiluted soup into a bowl. Add the garlic, salt and milk.
Plunk the mashed potatoes into a buttered casserole. Pour the cheese mixture over the top. Mix the bread crumbs with the melted butter and scatter over the top.
Shove the dish into a 350 oven for 30 minutes.

Beefy Potato Roast

6 medium potatoes
6 onions
1 teaspoon salt
  freshly ground black pepper
  olive oil
1 cup beef bouillon

Peel the potatoes and onions. Cut the potatoes into half-inch slices and the onions into quarter-inch slices. Mix in a bowl with the salt and pepper.
Grease an oven casserole with the oil. Layer the potatoes and onions, pour in the bouillon, cover the dish and shove into a 400-degree oven for 15 minutes.
Remove top of the casserole and continue to cook until the liquid has evaporated and the vegetables are tender and golden brown. Serves six.

A (cauli) Flower

3 cups cauliflower buds and chopped stems
1 tablespoon flour
¾ cup milk
¼ teaspoon salt
1/8 teaspoon cayenne pepper (or more)
1/8 teaspoon black pepper
1 teaspoon canola oil
½ cup shredded cheddar cheese
2 tablespoons chopped green chilies
1/3 cup bread crumbs

Steam the cauliflower over low heat just until tender. Do not overcook or Santa will leave a lump of chicken fat in your Christmas stocking. Drain and dump the veggies into an oven dish.
In a jar, shake together the flour, milk, salt, pepper and cayenne. When smooth, pour this muck into a saucepan containing the hot oil. Stir-cook until thickened, then stir in the cheese and chilies. When the cheese is melted, pour over the cauliflower, top with crumbs and bake in a 350-degree oven 10 to 15 minutes, until heated through. Serves four.

Cauliflower Curry

1 head cauliflower
1 onion, chopped
3 tablespoons butter
1 ½ tablespoon poppy seeds
1 ½ tablespoons curry powder
1 ½ teaspoons ground ginger
1 teaspoon cumin seed
¼ teaspoon hot pepper flakes
1 cup yogurt
1 package (10 ounces) frozen peas

Bring the peas to room temperature.
Core the cauliflower and cut the remainder into florets. Steam until tender but still crisp and drain. Remove to a warm dish.
Heat the butter in a skillet. Add the onion and stir-cook until it softens.
Add the poppy seed, curry powder, ginger, cumin and hot pepper flakes, stir-cooking for another minute.
Stir in the yogurt. Add the cauliflower and thawed peas, stir together to warm and serve immediately.

Cauliflower Ear

   1 head cauliflower
   ¼ cup butter
   ¼ cup slivered almonds
   2 tablespoons flour
   2 tablespoons minced parsley
   ½ cup chicken bouillon
   ½ cup white wine
   ½ cup sour cream
     Salt, pepper

   Cut the tough core of the vegetable away and steam the remaining cauliflower until barely done.
   Melt the butter in a skillet and saute the almonds until they begin to brown. Remove with a slotted spoon.
   Stir in the flour and parsley and stir-cook two minutes. Add the chicken bouillon and wine, and boil for one minute.
   Remove skillet from the heat and stir in the sour cream (yes you can use no-fat sour cream) and half the almonds. Add salt and pepper to taste.
   Pour this sludge over the cauliflower and sprinkle the remaining almonds over the top.

Green Bean Casserole for a Crowd

   2½ pounds fresh green beans
   ⅓ cup parsley, minced
   ½ teaspoon garlic powder
   1 teaspoon oregano
   ½ teaspoon celery seed
   ½ teaspoon basil
   ½ teaspoon pepper
   4 medium tomatoes, cut into thin wedges
   2 small onions, thinly sliced
   ½ cup grated Parmesan cheese
     butter

   Cook beans in boiling water until barely tender. Drain and mix with parsley and spices. Arrange half the beans in a large casserole. Arrange all the tomato wedges on top, then the onion rings. Top with half the cheese. Then dump in the rest of the beans, dot with butter and cover with the rest of the Parmesan. (Add more cheese if you think you need it and have a reputation as a big spender.) Shove casserole into a 350-degree oven for 25 minutes. Serves 18 to 20.

Red and Green Beans

   1 pound cooked green beans
   1½ tablespoon olive oil
   ¼ teaspoon salt
   1 sweet red pepper, cut in thin strips and cooked one minute
   2 tablespoons chopped toasted hazelnuts

   Toss all ingredients in a pan and serve to four customers when hot.

Zucchini Parmesan

   1 medium zucchini, unpeeled and chopped
   ¼ cup sour cream
   1 tablespoon butter
     Parmesan cheese
   ½ teaspoon salt
   ⅛ teaspoon paprika
   2 eggs, slightly beaten
     Buttered bread crumbs

   Simmer the chopped zucchini (you should have about 3 cups) in salted water for 6 or 7 minutes and drain. In a saucepan over low heat, combine the sour cream, butter, 2 tablespoons of Parmesan cheese, salt and paprika. Remove from the heat and stir in the egg or egg substitute.
   Combine this muck with the drained zucchini, plunk into a lightly oiled casserole and top with the buttered bread crumbs and more Parmesan. Bake 20 minutes in at 375 degrees.
   This will probably be enough zucchini to serve 4 as a side dish.

California Carrots

   4 carrots, quartered
   1 tablespoon sugar
   1 teaspoon cornstarch
   ¼ teaspoon salt
   ¼ teaspoon powdered ginger
   ¼ cup orange juice
   2 tablespoons butter or canola oil

   Cover carrots with water in a skillet and cook just until tender.
   Mix the sugar with the cornstarch, salt, ginger and orange juice. Heat and stir to thicken. Add butter or canola oil and pour over drained carrots. Serves 4.

Macaroni Veggies

    8 ounces macaroni
    3 tablespoons canola oil
    1 tablespoon flour
    ½ cup chicken stock
    ¾ cup skim milk
    1 cup grated cheddar cheese
    1 teaspoon dried basil
    ½ teaspoon paprika
    ¼ teaspoon black pepper
    2 cups broccoli florets and sliced stems
    1 sweet red pepper, coarsely chopped
    ½ pound fresh mushrooms, sliced
    3 green onions including green tops, chopped
       Cayenne pepper (optional)

Cook the macaroni in salted water according to directions on the package.

While the pasta water is splashing out of the pot onto the burner, heat 2 tablespoons oil in a saucepan, add the flour and stir until blended. Then whisk in the chicken broth and milk, stirring until it comes to a simmer and thickens. Reduce heat to low and stir in cheese and seasonings.

Drain the macaroni and let it sit in the colander for a minute while you heat the final tablespoon of oil in the same pot. Add the broccoli, red pepper and mushrooms, stirring, until the broccoli is barely done.

Toss in the macaroni and the cheese sauce, mix everything around and when it has reheated sufficiently serve to four hungry guests, scattering green onion bits over the top of each portion, along with cayenne pepper, to taste.

Another Veggie-Mac

    ⅔ cup diced carrots
    1 cup sliced cauliflower
    1 cup green beans, stringed and diced
    1 cup frozen peas, thawed
    8 ounces macaroni
    2 tablespoons olive oil
    ½ teaspoon dry mustard
    2½ tablespoons flour
    2 cups skim milk
    ½ tablespoon coriander
    4 ounces roasted red peppers from a jar, diced
    ¼ pound cheddar cheese, grated

Steam the carrots, cauliflower and green beans just until tender. Cook the macaroni in boiling, salted water until done. Drain and cover with cold water.

Grease a casserole dish and into it dump the veggies and the drained macaroni. Mix lightly with the hands.

Distribute the red peppers over the top.

Heat the oil in a saucepan. Add the flour and stir-cook 30 seconds. Add the milk and whisk, while cooking, until it thickens into sauce. Remove from the heat and add the coriander, mustard and one-quarter cup of the grated cheese.

Taste to see if it needs salt.

Pour all this over the veggies and macaroni and mix lightly. Sprinkle the rest of the cheese over the top and shove into a 375-degree oven for about 20 minutes, or until cheese has melted and the casserole ingredients are hot.

I like to add cajun spices to the sauce, but Alice likes it plain. So I sprinkle the spices over my portion after it's dished up.

This will serve four to six.

Stiragus

    1 pound fresh asparagus
    3 thin slices ginger root
    2 tablespoons canola oil
    ½ teaspoon salt
    ½ cup chicken broth
    1 tablespoons soy sauce
    ½ teaspoon sugar

Cut the tender tips off the asparagus and reserve. Cut the stalks into 1 ½ inch pieces. Drop the stalks into simmering water until barely tender. (Don't pre-cook the tips.)

Flatten then mince the ginger and heat in skillet with the oil and salt. After a minute add the asparagus tips and stalks. Stir once then add to the pan the broth, soy sauce and sugar. Cover and simmer two to three minutes, then serve hot to four guests.

Artichokes

    2 large artichokes
       salt
       non-fat sour cream
       low-fat mayonnaise
       Beau Monde seasoning
       dill weed

With a sharp knife cut off the stem of the chokes. Turn them around and slice off a half inch of the artichokes at the leaf end. Shove the artichokes into a snug pan and cover with water. Simmer covered just until the outside leaves will easily pull off. Let cool.

You can carve the artichoke in half to serve four. Or else serve one per customer.

Combine equal parts sour cream and mayonnaise and season with the Beau Monde and dill for an excellent dip.

Hungarian Cabbage

- 1 large head green cabbage
- 1 tablespoon salt
- 1/3 cup butter or canola oil
- 3 tablespoons sugar
- good grinding of black pepper

Don't have a cow over the amount of salt listed above. You are going to wash most of it away.

Traditionally this recipe is made with butter. I substitute the oil and sprinkle the cabbage liberally with Butter Buds when it is cooked.

OK, remove and discard the core and finely chop the cabbage. Mix the cabbage with the salt in a bowl and let stand 30 minutes. Then place cabbage in a colander and rinse briefly under cold water. Then squeeze out the liquid.

In a large skillet heat the butter or oil. Add the cabbage and cook over medium heat for 30 minutes, stirring occasionally. Stir in the sugar and pepper and continue cooking for another 15 minutes, or until the cabbage begins to brown. This will serve four.

Southern Greens

- 2 pounds greens (chard, kale etc.) stems removed
- 2 teaspoons olive oil
- 3 cloves minced garlic
- 1/4 teaspoon red pepper flakes
- Black pepper to taste
- 2 tablespoons lemon juice

Wash the greens, cut into 1-inch strips and toss (still wet) into a pot coated with olive oil. Add the garlic, red pepper flakes and black pepper.

Steam five minutes, remove and add lemon juice, plus salt if needed.

If half your guests are from Baton Rouge and the other half are from Soap Lake, you might want to go easy on the red pepper flakes (in the greens). Then you can pass the Tabasco at the table so the individual diners can decide how bad they want to burn their tongues.

Wayne's Spinach

- 2 pounds fresh spinach
- 3 green onions, chopped
- 1½ tablespoons butter
- 1½ tablespoons flour
- 1 cup milk
- 3 tablespoons fat-free sour cream
- ½ teaspoon nutmeg
- 1 teaspoon lemon juice
- ¼ cup freshly grated Parmesan

Wash the spinach, discarding heavy stems. Place wet leaves in an empty saucepan and steam, covered, using only the water that clings to them. Stir once or twice. The spinach should be wilted after 4 or 5 minutes. Drain, then spray with cold water.

In your fist, wring the water out of the spinach and puree it in a food processor or blender.

Melt the butter in another small pan and add the green onions. Cook slowly for a minute, then stir in the flour. When it has mixed into the butter, slowly add the milk and stir until it thickens into a sauce.

In a mixing bowl, combine the spinach, the white sauce, sour cream, nutmeg, lemon juice and salt to taste. Stir in the Parmesan.

Transfer to a small casserole and heat in a 350-degree oven for 20 minutes.

Beta Carotene Sources

- ✿ Sweet potatoes
- ✿ Spinach
- ✿ Pumpkin
- ✿ Squash
- ✿ Carrots
- ✿ Collard Greens
- ✿ Cantaloupe
- ✿ Apricots

Vitamin E Sources

- ✿ Peanuts
- ✿ Sunflower seeds, oil
- ✿ Peanut butter
- ✿ Wheat germ
- ✿ Mayonnaise
- ✿ Safflower oil

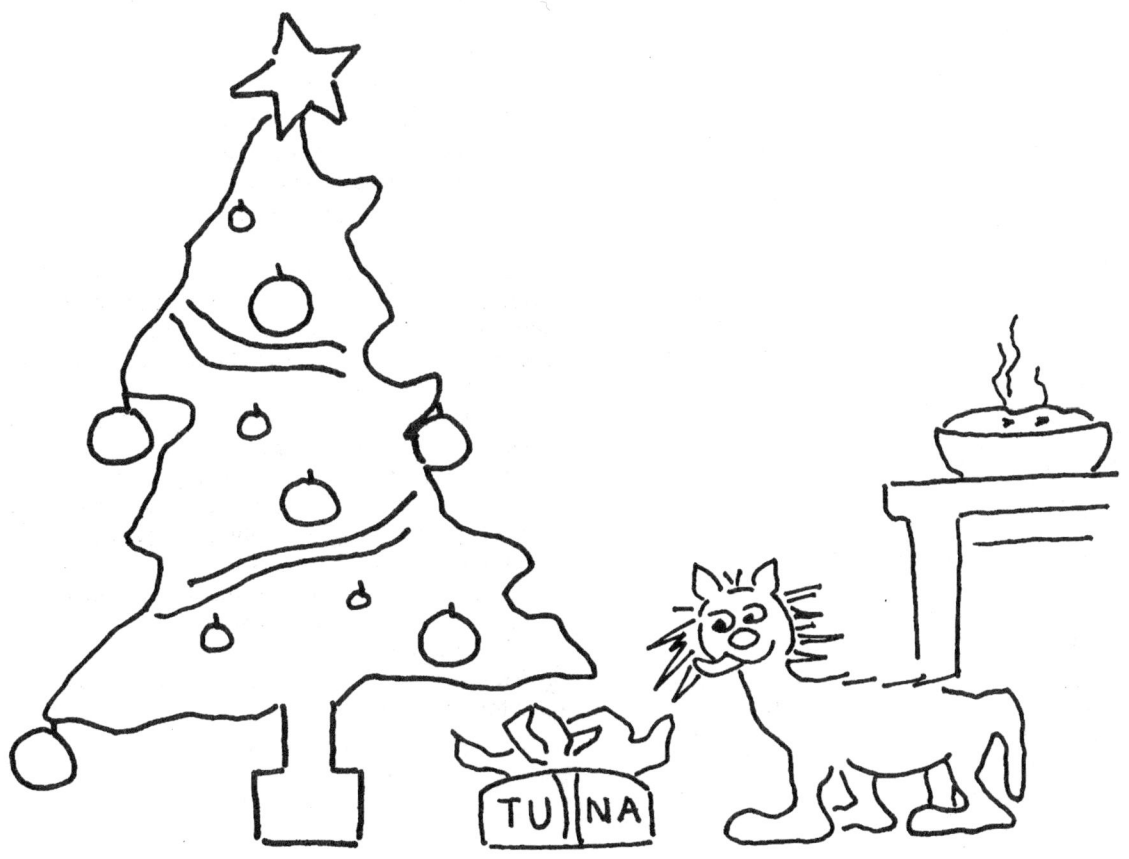

CASSEROLES

In this instance only, you are allowed to open your present before Christmas.

Maybe you already guessed what it was. Even with silver wrapping paper and a large red bow, it's hard to disguise a can of tuna. Trying to gift-wrap some Omega-3 fatty acids is an even greater challenge.

See, I'm giving you much more than the ingredients for next week's sack lunch. You're also getting good health and an answer to the annual question: What do you serve the family on Christmas Eve when your Visa card is setting off burglar alarms in all the local markets?

Recent preventive medicine studies indicate Omega-3 is a greater boon to health than an electric vitamin dispenser. And what are the three best sources of Omega-3? Black cod, salmon and albacore tuna. I was considering putting a half-pound codfish steak under your Christmas tree but I figured the cat would have it unwrapped and eaten before you could utter, "Ho, ho, ho!"

But that's not necessary. The fountain of youth is located in a 6-ounce can. The secret to good health and long life is the long-maligned tuna casserole. What's more, I've got the formula for a couple that actually taste good and will feed Santa and most of his elves.

Christmas Eve Casserole

    1 tablespoon olive oil
    2 cans tuna
    1 can (8 ounces) mushrooms
    1 clove garlic
    1 bay leaf
    1 teaspoon anchovy paste (optional)
    1 teaspoon salt
    ½ teaspoon dry basil
    1 teaspoon Tabasco sauce
    1 large can (16 ounces) tomato sauce
    8 ounces noodles or spaghetti
    2 packages (10 ounces each) chopped frozen spinach
    ½ cup grated Parmesan cheese

Cook and squeeze-dry the spinach. Cook the noodles in salted boiling water and drain.

OK, heat the oil in a large skillet. Drain the mushrooms, saving the liquid. Dump the mushrooms and chopped garlic into the pan and saute 5 minutes. Add the bay leaf, anchovy paste, basil, salt and tomato sauce and simmer 10 minutes. Remove the bay leaf and add to the pan the tuna (I use albacore) and the Tabasco. Cook another 5 minutes.

Place half the cooked noodles in a casserole. Top with half the spinach and half the sauce. Repeat layers and top with Parmesan cheese.

Heat the casserole in a 350-degree oven for 30 minutes, or until bubbling hot.

Tuna-Mushroom Hot Dish

    8 ounces dried, broad noodles
    1 tablespoon margarine
    ½ cup chopped onion
    1 6-ounce can mushrooms stems and pieces
    ¼ teaspoon celery salt
    ½ teaspoon dill weed
    1 tablespoon sherry
    1 can golden mushroom soup
    ¼ cup skim milk
    1/3 cup grated Parmesan cheese
    2 cans (14 ounces total) chunk tuna
    1 cup frozen peas
        Dry bread crumbs
        Creole seasoning or cayenne pepper

Cook the noodles according to package instructions. Drain in a colander, then cool under running water.

In the noodle pan heat the margarine and add the onion. Saute until soft, then add the mushrooms, celery salt, dill weed, sherry, undiluted soup, the skim milk and the cheese. Stir to mix, then fold in the tuna and peas.

Plunk the noodles into a greased casserole. Top with the mushroom-tuna mixture and combine gently with two forks.

Scatter some bread crumbs over the top and sprinkle with Creole seasoning or with a bit of cayenne pepper.

Shove into a 350-degree oven for 25 minutes; this should serve four.

This dish is also good with leftover salmon replacing the tuna. Or you can combine tuna and salmon in the same casserole.

Wild Turkey Casserole

    1 cup minute brown rice
    1½ cups salted water
    3 tablespoons toasted sunflower seeds
    ½ pound Jimmy Dean Lite sausage
    1/3 pound fresh mushrooms
    1 can cream of mushroom soup
    1 pound leftover turkey, cubed

Cook the rice in salted water according to package instructions. Drain and stir in the sunflower seeds. Toss the sausage into the skillet along with the sliced mushrooms. Bust meat up with wooden spoon.

Remove from heat when the sausage is lightly browned. Pour off any fat. Dump half the cooked rice into the bottom of a buttered casserole, top with half the sausage-mushroom mixture, half the turkey and then gloop in half the undiluted soup. Repeat the layers, cover and bake 30 minutes in a 375-degree oven.

Healthy Oils

The following oils all have high percentages of monounsaturated fats, which is preferable in almost all cases.

- Avocado oil
- Cashew oil
- Olive oil
- Peanut oil
- Canola oil

The Bad Oils

- Coconut
- Palm

Read the ingredients of baked goods and processed foods and try to avoid anything containing either of these oils. Products containing cotton seed oils should also be avoided.

Seafood Italian

  1 can (4 ½ ounces) tuna
  ½ pound fresh, small shrimp
  ½ cup chopped onion
  ½ of a green pepper, seeded and chopped
  3 tablespoons canola oil
  3 tablespoons flour
      Chicken broth
  ½ teaspoon crushed fennel seed
  ½ teaspoon celery seed
  1 teaspoon pepper
      Splat of Tabasco
  1 tablespoon sherry
      Salt to taste
  ¼ cup grated Parmesan cheese
  8 ounces penne pasta, cooked and drained

Saute the onions and green pepper in the oil. Add flour and stir-cook over low heat five minutes. Pour the liquid from the tuna can into a measuring cup. Add chicken broth to achieve a cup and a half of liquid. Stir this into the flour-veggie mess and bring to a boil to thicken.

Remove the sauce from the heat and add remaining ingredients. Spoon into a greased casserole, top with more Parmesan if you are a really, really big spender. And bake about 45 minutes in a 300-degree oven. This should serve four to six.

Swiss and Spinach

  8 ounces small tube pasta
  ¼ cup Canola oil
  ¼ cup flour
  2 cups milk
 12 ounces Swiss cheese
  ½ teaspoon Tabasco sauce
  1 tablespoon Dijon mustard
  ½ pound ham, in thin strips
  1 package (10 ounces) frozen spinach
      Salt and pepper

Thaw the spinach and shred the cheese while softly humming the soundtrack from a silent film.

Cook the pasta, drain and let sit in cold water.

Heat the oil in a large pan, stir in the flour and when this mess begins to bubble add the milk.

Keep stirring until the muck has thickened, then add two-thirds of the cheese, the Tabasco and mustard. Remove from heat.

Drain the pasta and mix with the cheese sauce. Stir in the ham strips.

Squeeze out excess moisture from the spinach and mix that in, too.

Dump everything into a casserole, top with the last of the cheese and cook in a 325-degree oven until bubbly.

Van Gogh's Paella

  1 fryer chicken, cut up
  2 garlic cloves, minced
  4 green onions, chopped
  ¼ cup olive oil
  ¼ pound Jimmy Dean Lite sausage meat
  2 tomatoes, chopped
  1 package (10 ounces) frozen peas
  1 (8 ounce) can artichoke hearts, quartered
  2 teaspoons paprika
 1½ cups raw rice
  1 teaspoon salt
  4 cups chicken broth
 12 pimento olives
 12 peeled shrimp
 24 or more steamer clams

Instead of a whole chicken, you can use an equivalent amount of chicken thighs. Pour some oil in your paella pan or skillet and brown the seasoned chicken pieces. Remove.

Toss the garlic, onions and sausage meat into the pan. When the onion has softened, add the tomatoes, peas, artichoke hearts, paprika and rice. Cook until the rice is well coated with oil, then add the broth; salt if needed.

Simmer uncovered until rice is almost tender and most of the liquid has cooked away. Arrange shrimp, olives and cooked chicken atop the rice.

Meanwhile, in another pot, steam the clams in ½ cup water (or dry vermouth) until they open.

When the shrimp are pink and the paella is done, top with the clams and pour the clam nectar over the rice, too. Serves six.

Don't Blame It On the Cows

An eight-ounce glass of whole milk contains 8.5 grams of fat. Here are some healthier alternatives.

Two per cent milk .... 5.3 grams fat

One per cent milk .... 2.5 grams fat

Skim milk .... Half of one per cent fat

Blended Scotch Whiskey . . . No fat, but it tastes terrible on Grape Nuts.

No-Neurosis Enchiladas

- ¼ cup canola oil
- ¼ cup flour
- 2 cups chicken broth
- 1 cup yogurt
- 1 can (7 ounces) mild chopped chilies
- 12 corn tortillas (6 inches wide)
- 2 cups cooked chicken
- 1 small onion, chopped
- 12 ounces cheese, grated (jack or low-fat Velveeta)
- ¼ cup green onions, chopped

Heat the oil in a pot, then stir in the flour. After it has cooked for a minute whisk in the broth and stir until boiling. Remove from the heat and add the yogurt and chilies.

Cover the bottom of a 9-by-12-inch oven dish with one-third of the sauce.

Quickly dip the tortillas in water. Drain quickly and cut into 1-inch strips. Scatter half of the tortillas strips over the sauce. Cover with chicken, onion, two-thirds of the cheese and one-third of the sauce. Make another layer with the rest of the tortilla strips, sauce and cheese.

Cover the dish with foil and bake 30 to 35 minutes at 400 degrees. Sprinkle with green onions.

This will serve 6 to 8 people. But because it isn't swimming in fat, it needs a jolt of flavor – and this sauce provides it:

Special Salsa

- 1 ripe tomato, chopped
- 3 green onions, minced
- ¼ cup minced cilantro
- 1 clove garlic, minced
- 2 jalapeno peppers from a jar, chopped
- ½ teaspoon salt
- ¼ teaspoon sugar
- ⅓ cup fresh lime juice

Combine all these ingredients shortly before you will need the sauce. Let your guests spoon the mixture over their individual portions of enchiladas.

The sauce is easy to make but deteriorates in the refrigerator after a day or two.

A Near-East Feast

- 2 whole chicken breasts
- 2¾ cups chicken stock
- 2 medium onions
- 3 tablespoons cooking oil
- 2 cloves garlic
- 2 tablespoons curry powder
- 1 teaspoon ground cumin
- 1 teaspoon salt
- 2 teaspoons ground ginger
- ½ teaspoon ground cloves
- ½ teaspoon ground cinnamon
- ½ teaspoon black pepper
- 1½ cups uncooked rice
- 2 packages frozen chopped spinach

Let the spinach thaw at room temperature.

Separate the breasts so you have four pieces. Dump them in a pan and cover with water. Bring to a boil, remove from heat and let sit about 10 minutes until they are lightly poached.

Cut chicken into bite-sized pieces and don't worry if some seem underdone. They will get a second cooking in the oven.

Chop the onions and saute in oil. Combine in a bowl the curry, cumin, salt, ginger, cloves, cinnamon, pepper and minced garlic. When the onions have softened, add all the ingredients of the bowl and stir-cook with the onions for three or four minutes.

Plunk the chicken hunks into a casserole. Scatter the rice over the top.

Then make another layer out of the spiced onions. Pour the chicken stock over the rice.

Finally, squeeze the spinach lightly to remove some of the liquid then spread it over the top of the casserole.

Cover the casserole and shove into a preheated, 375-degree oven. Cook just until the rice is done, probably about 40 minutes, removing from the oven once or twice to test. If you like your curry jazzed up a bit, you can top your portion with chopped green onions, peanuts, coconut or with a bit of chutney on the side.

This should serve at least four.

Sources of Omega-3

- Mackerel
- Herring
- Black cod
- Tuna
- Salmon
- Sablefish
- Anchovy
- Lake trout
- Shark
- Oysters
- Mussels
- Dog fish

As a rule of thumb, the colder the water inhabited by the fish, the more Omega-3 fats it contains.

Macaroni and Cheese

- ¾ pound dried macaroni
- 3 tablespoons butter or canola oil
- 2 tablespoons flour
- 4 cups milk
- 1 tablespoon Dijon mustard
- salt to taste
- ½ teaspoon nutmeg
- 1/8 teaspoon cayenne pepper
- 1 onion, chopped
- ¼ pound fresh mushrooms, sliced
- ½ pound ham, cubed
- 2½ cups cheddar cheese

Cook the pasta and then immerse in cold water.

In a saucepan heat two tablespoons of butter (or oil) until sizzling. Stir in the flour and cook for a minute. Slowly stir in three cups of milk. Stir as it thickens then add the mustard, nutmeg, cayenne and salt. Remove from heat.

In a skillet heat the final tablespoon of butter. Saute the onions until soft. Add the mushrooms and ham and cook another five minutes.

Return the sauce to the heat and add the cheese, grated or cubed. When it has melted stir in the ham-mushroom mess.

At this point decide if the sauce needs to be thinned. If so, add all or part of the final cup of milk. This dish is best made with a medium cheddar but if you are cutting back on calories you can substitute low-fat Velvetta and skim milk. The sauce will be OK, but might not need as much liquid and probably could use a bit more cayenne to give it a bite.

OK, drain the macaroni and spoon half of it into a buttered casserole. Slop half the sauce over the top, top with the remaining macaroni and the rest of the sauce. If you think it is still a bit sloppy for your taste sprinkle some Italian bread crumbs over the top.

In any event, shove the casserole into a 400-degree oven for 20 minutes and it should serve four.

Asparachick

- 8 to 10 boned and skinned chicken thighs
- 2 chicken bouillon cubes
- ¼ cup chopped carrots
- handful of celery tops
- 4 tablespoons butter (or canola oil)
- 4 tablespoons flour
- 1 cup cream (or low-fat evaporated milk)
- 2 tablespoons sherry
- 2 cups cooked spaghetti
- ½ pound trimmed but uncooked asparagus
- 4 tablespoons Parmesan cheese
- 1 cup seasoned dry bread crumbs

Toss the chicken thighs into a pot and cover with water. Add the carrots and celery tops, bring water to a boil, then turn off heat and let sit for an hour.

Remove the thighs and when cool cut each into two or three pieces. Strain the hot broth, reserving two cups. Add two bouillon cubes.

Heat the butter or oil in a saucepan. Stir in the flour and stir-cook one minute. Slowly add the two cups of chicken broth, stirring until smooth. Add the cream and reheat but do not boil. Finally, add the sherry and remove from heat.

Lay the cooked spaghetti out in a greased casserole. Top with a layer of asparagus, then the chicken and finally cover with the sauce, the grated Parmesan cheese and top with the bread crumbs.

Shove the dish into a 325-degree oven for 30 minutes. Serves four or more.

The Perfect Non-Fattening Product

Tell the waiter to, "Make mine water." An intake of six to eight glasses of water a day is recommended. For starters, you may not notice the hunger pangs as much if your stomach is awash. But water is also essential for those trying to increase the fiber in their diet, since it speeds the digestive process.

Remember, we're not talking about six to eight glasses of fluids. Tea coffee, soft drinks, beer and soft drinks don't count. Caffeine and alcohol can cause dehydration. That's something your favorite bartender, or espresso dispenser, never told you.

Ham-Noodle Casserole

    10 ounces dry noodles
     2 tablespoons canola oil
     2 cups diced ham
    ¼   cup onions, minced
     1 green pepper, seeded and cubed
     1 clove garlic, minced
     1 cup chopped tomatoes
     1 4- to 6-ounce can sliced mushrooms
     1 6-ounce can tomato sauce
     1 teaspoon curry powder
     1 cup frozen peas
        Salt and black pepper
        Cayenne pepper
        Cheddar cheese

Cook noodles in salted water, then drain.

While the noodles are cooking, heat the oil in a skillet. Add the ham, onions, green pepper and garlic. Cook 2 minutes, then dump in the tomatoes, mushrooms with liquid and the curry powder.

Plunk the noodles in a casserole and mix in the ingredients of the skillet. Stir in the tomato sauce and peas. Taste to see how much salt, pepper and cayenne it needs and add accordingly.

Grate enough cheddar cheese to cover the top.

Bake the casserole 30 minutes or until bubbling in a 350-degree oven.

This should serve four to six residents of Sand Coulee, Mont.

Cross-Country Casserole

    1¼ pounds lean ground turkey
     1 clove garlic, minced
     2 green peppers, seeded and chopped
     1 large onion, peeled and chopped
     1 tablespoon chili powder
     2 teaspoons paprika
     2 teaspoons salt
    ½   teaspoon dried oregano, crumbled
     1 can (16 ounces) chopped tomatoes
     1 can (8 ounce) tomato sauce
     2 tablespoons barbecue sauce (or ketchup)
     8 ounces noodles
    1½ cups grated cheddar or American cheese
     8 green olives (optional)

Brown the turkey in a heavy pot. You may need a bit of oil if it is extra lean. After 3 minutes of stirring and busting up the meat with a wooden spoon, toss the garlic, chopped peppers and onion into the pot and cook another 4 minutes, stirring occasionally.

Stir in the chili powder, paprika, salt, oregano, tomatoes, tomato sauce and barbecue sauce. Simmer this mess over medium heat for 15 minutes.

Cook the noodles in salted, boiling water. Drain thoroughly, then dump the noodles into the pot with the tomato sauce. Stir, then transfer the whole works to an oven casserole. Top with the grated cheese.

If you are traveling first cabin on this flight, top the cheese with the pimento green olives, sliced.

Shove the casserole into a preheated, 350-degree oven for 20 to 30 minutes.

This should serve 1 wolf or 4-6 cross-country skiers.

Bringing Up The Rear In the Great Poultry Hunt

The Intermediate Eater tends to favor chicken thighs, rather than breasts, in casserole dishes. It's a personal prejudice. Dark meat doesn't dry out as fast and tends to be more flavorful.

But if you need to cut your fat quotient to the bone, you probably should substitute white meat, shortening the cooking process by a few minutes.

There is a big difference in fat content. Dark meat, from drumstick or thigh, has about twice as much fat per ounce as white breast meat.

However, leaving the skin on doubles the fat content of chicken breast and triples the fat in a portion of turkey breast.

If you are cooking a full chicken, the combination of white and dark meat is usually a healthier option than even the leanest red meats. Remove the skin from the chicken after cooking, if you are roasting a full bird. Remove it before oven cooking pieces of thigh or breast. To obtain meat for a casserole, poach the chicken in water.

In parts of the American south, some gourmands prefer to deep fry whole chickens or turkeys in oil drums filled with hot lard. In some parts of northern Russia they play roulette with loaded pistols, and chase shots of 100 proof vodka with bites of dill pickle. None of these options is endorsed by the American Medical Association.

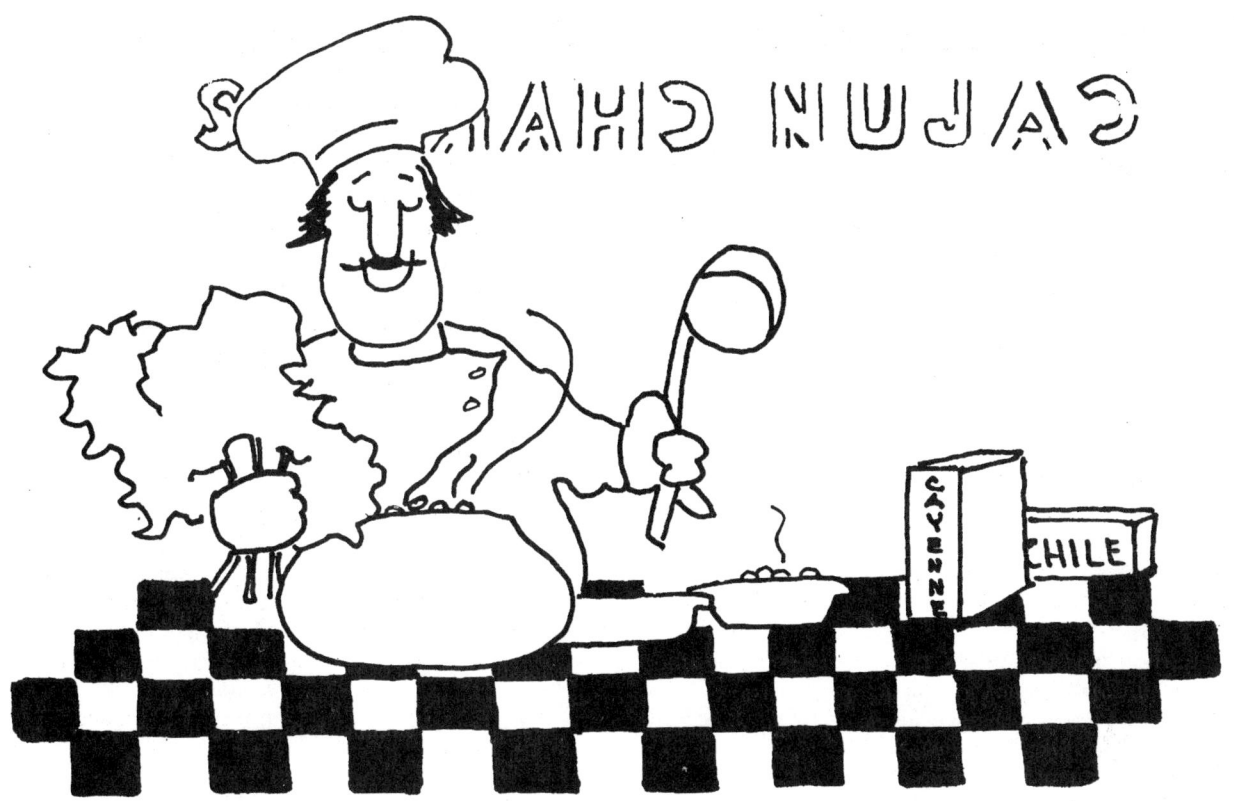

BEANS AND RICE

Just suppose there was a magic black pill that would supply your body with protein, carbohydrates, iron, magnesium, zinc and folacin. And suppose there was a magic white pill high in vitamin B, rich in calcium and iron.

And suppose your nutritional adviser told you that the black pill enhances the white pill and together they create the almost perfect food. It's true.

And the nutritional value is even higher if the black and white pills are served with some tomatoes, peppers and ham.

Don't ask me why, because the explanation involves a lot of tryptophan, methionine, ferrous iron, phytic acid and tends to give me a nagging headache.

All you really have to know is that the white pills are grains of rice, the black pills are beans, and I've got a terrific recipe combining both. So does every native of Miami, New Orleans, Tuscaloosa, Havana and Possum Trot.

In Louisiana you probably will be served a variation of red beans and rice.

In Florida or the Caribbean, it will likely be black beans and rice.

"Doan make no differnts," the local residents would advise you. Served up with a side dish of boiled greens and pot liquor and you have a fuel capable of rocketing a wagon full of Cajuns to the moon and back.

An equivalent meal in Seattle might carry you only to Nooksack and back, because local chefs tend to be timid with chili powder and cayenne pepper. But it's still a great meal, nutritionally and astronomically. And you build it according to the specifications listed on the next page.

Black Beans and Rice

    Canola oil
3 cloves garlic, minced
1 medium onion, chopped
1 teaspoon ground cumin
1 teaspoon chili powder
1 slice ham (quarter pound)
1 sweet green pepper, chopped
2 15-ounce cans black beans
1 14-ounce can chopped tomatoes
½ cup tomato or V8 juice
    salt, pepper to taste
    cayenne pepper
2 cups raw rice
    Sour cream
    Chopped green onions

    Heat enough canola oil to cover the bottom of a skillet. Toss in the onion, garlic, cumin, chili powder, the green pepper and the ham, diced. Cook over medium heat four or five minutes, stirring occasionally.

    Drain one can of beans and add to the skillet. Add the other can of beans, undrained. Then toss in the tomatoes, with the can juices. Add the tomato or V8 juice as needed when the pan juices cook down.

    Reduce heat to a simmer and taste to see how much salt, pepper and cayenne you want to add. You want this dish to be fairly spicy.

    While the beans are simmering, bring a large pot of water to a boil. Add two teaspoons of salt to the water then stir in the rice. Let rice boil 12 minutes, then drain through a large strainer. Heap the drained rice in a bowl and fluff with a fork.

    Put the skillet mixture on the table, along with the rice. Let everybody spoon up a mountain of rice, cover with beans and top with sour cream and chopped green onions.

    If you are emphasizing nutrition over taste, you can use nonfat sour cream.

    Or you can leave it off altogether.

    This will serve four or more with southern greens (see chapter on Vegetables.)

Is It Really "Low Fat?"

    Buy ground beef with less than 10 per cent fat. If it isn't marked for fat content, don't buy it.
    Ground turkey should have a fat content of 7 per cent or less.

All-Day Cassoulet

1 can (1 pound) red kidney beans
1 can (1 pound) garbanzo beans
1 can (1 pound) black-eyed peas
¼ teaspoon thyme
¼ teaspoon black pepper
2 large onions
½ pound lean pork
4 tablespoons olive oil
1 cup dry white wine
6 small, low-fat sausage links

    When your Felix the Cat alarm radio goes off, pour beans into a large bowl and add the thyme and pepper. Transfer to an oven casserole. Quarter the peeled onions and sink them into the beans. Cover the casserole and bake in a 225-degree oven for two hours.

    Cut pork and the sausages into small pieces and brown in a skillet with hot oil. Add the wine and simmer, covered, for 10 minutes.

    With a slotted spoon add the meat to the beans. Pour in just enough of the wine from the pan to barely show through the beans. Cover casserole and return to the oven for another hour. Add salt and pepper to taste. Serves six.

Wild Bill's Beans

1 pound dried lima beans
1 onion, peeled and chopped
1 can (14 ounces) peeled and chopped tomatoes
2 tablespoons cooking oil
2 cloves garlic, minced
½ teaspoon ground sage or 2 tablespoons fresh
¾ pound ham, in chunks
    Black pepper

    Cover beans with water, bring to a boil for two minutes, remove from heat and let sit for an hour covered. Drain the water. Add fresh water and two teaspoons of salt. Cook until tender and drain again. Don't overcook the beans or they'll become mooshy, which is worse than mushy.

    Heat the oil in a pot and saute the onion and garlic. Add the beans and all the other ingredients except the pepper. Pour on boiling water to barely cover the beans.

    Bake in a 350-degree oven for 20 minutes, covered. Remove lid and bake 40 minutes more. Add lots of freshly ground pepper and announce to all those famished ranch hands that, "there is one item which does not appear on the regular menu tonight..."

Pipeline Beans

　　3　green onions
　　½　green pepper, chopped
　　½　cup chopped ham
　　2　tablespoons butter or canola oil
　　1　6-ounce can tomato paste
　　1　cup dry red wine
　　2　16-ounce cans kidney beans
　　½　teaspoon Italian seasonings
　　¼　cup Parmesan cheese
　　2　strips bacon (optional)

　　Heat the butter or oil in a pan. Chop the green onions, tops and all, and toss them into the pan along with the green pepper and ham. After a couple of minutes add the tomato paste and wine. Simmer 5 minutes.
　　Dump in the drained kidney beans, Italian seasonings, salt and pepper to taste and the grated Parmesan cheese.
　　Plop into an oven casserole, top with the two strips of bacon and bake at 350 degrees for 30 minutes. This will serve five. Leave off the bacon, if you want to reduce the fat content.

Mexican Beans

　　2　pounds black beans
　　4　teaspoons salt
　　2　onions, chopped
　　4　sweet peppers - red, green or combined - chopped
　　4　cloves garlic, put through a press
　　2　tablespoons ground cumin
　　　　Olive oil
　　1　small can tomato paste
　　3　tablespoons red wine vinegar
　　½　cup chopped green onions
　　½　cup minced cilantro leaves
　　　　Salt, black pepper and cayenne pepper

　　Soak the beans in water for an hour. Drain, cover again, drain again, then dump into a large pot.
　　Cover the beans with water by 1 inch and simmer uncovered until tender.
　　This will take 1 to 2 hours and you should have a pot of hot water standing by. Whenever the water covering the beans has boiled away, add more so the beans will always be covered. When they are tender add the salt and cook another 5 minutes.
　　Meanwhile, saute the onions, sweet peppers, garlic and cumin in olive oil until the vegetables are soft. Stir in the tomato paste and vinegar, simmer 2 minutes then stir this mess into the beans.
　　Add more salt, black pepper and cayenne pepper to taste.
　　Scatter green onions and cilantro over the top before plunking the pot on the buffet table.

Beanareeno

　　1　can (16 ounces) baked beans
　　1　can (16 ounces) kidney beans
　　1　can (16 ounces) pinto beans
　　1　green pepper, chopped
　　3　green onions, chopped
　　1　can (16 ounces) chopped tomatoes
　　1　package (1 ½ ounces) Sloppy Joe seasoning mix
　　½　cup shredded cheddar cheese

　　Drain the kidney and pinto beans and plunk into an oven dish. Add the baked beans, undrained, plus the green pepper, tomatoes, onion, and the seasoning mix. Scatter the cheese over the top and shove the casserole into a 350-degree oven until bubbling (30 to 40 minutes). Serves six or more.

Cable Car Rice

　　1　onion, chopped
　　¼　cup butter or canola oil
　　1　cup rice
　　2　cups chicken broth
　　　　Salt, pepper and oregano to taste

　　In a pot, saute the onion in butter or oil until soft and translucent. Add rice and stir until it begins to darken. Add the broth, stir pot, then cover and simmer. After 15 minutes check to see if the rice is done. If not, continue to steam until it is. Add salt, pepper and oregano to taste.

Capt. Cook's Rice

　　1　cup brown or wild rice
　　　　(or combination of the two)
　　⅓　cup chopped onions
　　½　cup diced celery
　　1　10-ounce can beef bouillon
　　1⅔　cans water
　　1　teaspoon salt (or to taste)
　　¼　cup butter, cut in bits
　　1　cup green stuffed olives, halved
　　½　cup grated Parmesan cheese

　　Plunk the rice, onions, celery, bouillon, water and salt into a greased, shallow casserole. Dot top with butter and bake uncovered in a 350-degree oven for 45 minutes. Mix in olives, top with cheese and bake another 15 minutes.
　　Serves the skipper, two sailors and one angry dockworker with a sore thumb.

Ginger Fried Rice

    1 cup white rice
    ½ teaspoon salt
    2½ tablespoons Canola oil
    2 teaspoons peeled and grated ginger root
    ⅔ cup frozen peas, thawed
    ⅔ cup frozen corn, thawed
    ½ cup grated carrot
    4 green onions, sliced
    1 teaspoon Worcestershire sauce
    4 teaspoons basil vinegar
    ½ cup chopped parsley

For recipes like this, keep in your refrigerator some peeled ginger root in a small bottle, covered with sherry. If you don't have basil vinegar, add a pinch of dried basil to white wine vinegar.

OK, wash the rice while you are bringing a cup and a half of water to a boil in a saucepan. Add to the water the rice and salt, lower heat and simmer the rice, covered, for 18 minutes or until done. Let it cool in a bowl for at least half an hour.

At dinner time heat the oil in a large skillet. Add the ginger and stir-cook 30 seconds at a medium-hot temperature. Add the rice and vegetables and stir-cook for 2 minutes. Mix the vinegar with the Worcestershire and slop this mess into the rice mixture. Stir-cook another minute, stir in the parsley and taste to see if some salt and pepper are needed. This will serve four.

Multiply the recipe if you plan to serve it at a luau, a wedding reception or at the annual North Dakota picnic and thaw-out in Hanauma Bay Park.

Hoover Hazelnut Rice

    2 tablespoons butter
    ½ cup chopped celery
    ½ cup chopped onion
    2½ cups chicken broth
    1 teaspoon salt, or to taste
    1 cup uncooked brown rice
    ½ cup chopped hazelnuts

Saute the celery and onion in butter until soft. Add broth and bring to a boil. Add the rice and salt. Cover pot, reduce heat and simmer 40 to 50 minutes or until tender. Add the hazelnuts.

This should serve four to six.

3 B Casserole

    ¼ cup butter
    ⅓ cup chopped almonds
    1 medium onion, chopped
    1 large carrot, peeled and chopped
    1 clove garlic, pressed
    ⅓ cup barley
    ⅓ cup brown rice
    ⅓ cup bulgar wheat (Ala)
    2½ cups chicken broth
    ¼ cup sherry
    ½ teaspoon salt (or to taste)
    2 tablespoons chopped sage leaves (or 1 teaspoon dried)
    ⅓ cup chopped parsley

In a large skillet melt the butter and briefly saute the nuts. Remove and add to the pan the onion, carrot and garlic. Saute 3 minutes, then add the grains. Cook another 3 minutes.

Add to the pan the broth, sherry, salt and sage. Bring to a boil then simmer, covered, 45 minutes.

Turn off the heat and let sit another 10 minutes then stir in the nuts and parsley and this should serve four to six cowpokes, sheep herders or sod busters.

Olympia Wild Rice

    2 cups of water
    2 teaspoons chicken bouillon powder
    ⅔ cup wild rice
    1 teaspoon salt
    4 tablespoons butter
    ⅔ cup minced carrot
    ⅔ cup chopped onion
    4 tablespoons minced parsley

Combine water, bouillon and rice in saucepan. Bring to a boil and simmer 45 minutes, or until rice has absorbed the liquid.

In a skillet cook the carrots in butter. Add the onion and cook 5 minutes.

Remove the skillet from the heat, stir in the wild rice and parsley, and serve as a side dish to four guests.

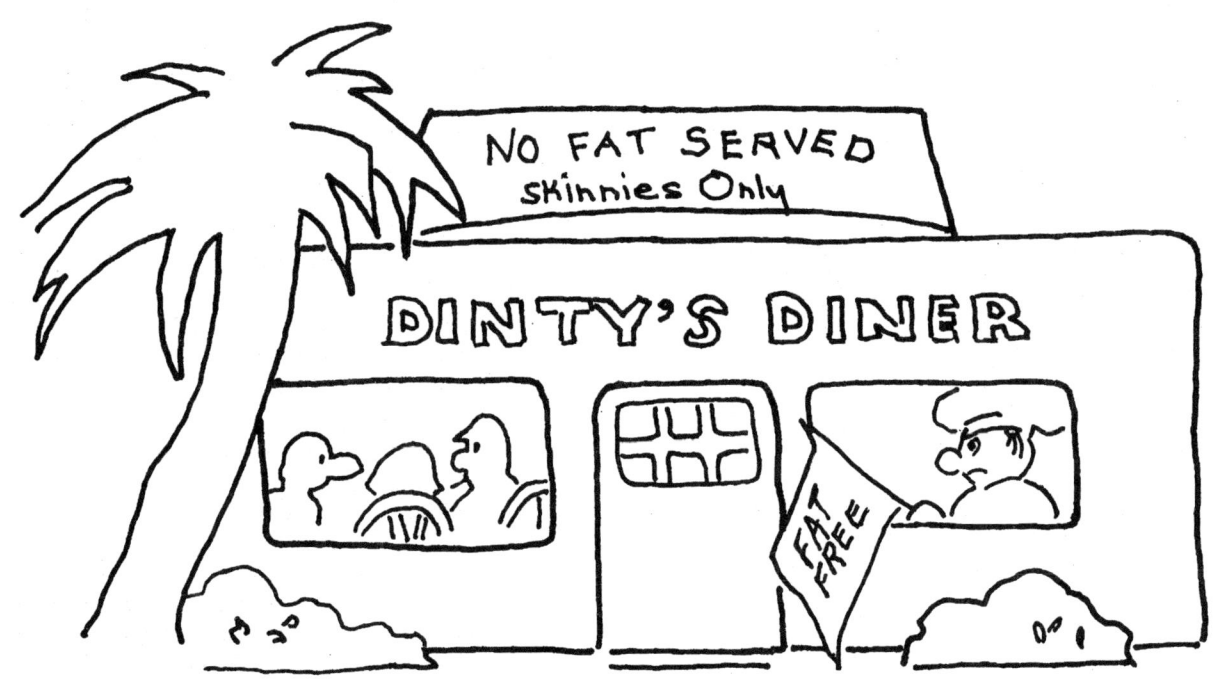

APPETIZERS

Let it be recorded for the edification of future historians. It was in the year 1994 that the Skinnies won the war. During that same 12-month span the Forces of Fat pulled down their colors, then reluctantly raised a white flag.

The surrender document was initialed by Jimmy Dean. In place of ink, he signed with melted Velveeta cheese.

For years we have been hearing about The New American Diet, high in oat bran and veggies, low in cholesterol and saturated fats. Yet if you walked into a typical American diner on a Sunday morning, you could not help but notice that most of the visitors were putting away four-egg omelets oozing with cheese. Included were side orders of hash browns crisped in the fat of the bacon that also rested on the enormous breakfast platters.

People talked thin. But they ate fat.

All that began to change in 1994. Who told me? Jimmy Dean. And those Kraft executives identified as members of the Velveeta Vatican.

Check it out. It was in 1994 that both Jimmy Dean sausage and Velveeta cheese appeared on the grocery shelves with low-fat products. The package labels suggest that the sausage and the cheese, combined, contain less saturated fat than a Spaulding tennis ball.

OK, purists may insist that Velveeta is not really a cheese, in either of its forms. And pig farmers may argue that Jimmy Dean's low-fat breakfast meat is not really sausage, since most of the pork has been replaced by lean turkey meat.

But the new products were enthusiastically welcomed by the Intermediate Eater. Because once again, with a clear conscience, I can enjoy my favorite cocktail snack which you will discover when you flip the next page.

New Age Sausage Snack

- 1 package (12 oz.) Jimmy Dean low-fat sage sausage
- 1 pound low-fat Velveeta, in hunks
- 1 pound extra lean ground beef
- 1 chopped onion
- 1 tablespoon Worcestershire sauce
- ½ teaspoon garlic salt
- ½ teaspoon oregano
- 2 tablespoons minced parsley
- Cocktail rye bread

Plop the sausage, onion and ground beef in a lightly oiled skillet and saute until brown. Add the cheese and all the other ingredients. When the cheese has melted you're in business.

Spread the glunk on the small cocktail rye rounds, place on a cookie sheet and bake for eight minutes in a 450-degree oven.

This makes a bunch of glunk but the prepared cocktail rye canapes can be kept almost indefinitely in a freezer, wrapped, then baked when needed without thawing.

Jungle Dip

- 13 ounces of chopped black olives
- 1 bunch green onions, chopped
- 1 7-ounce can chopped green chilies
- ¾ cup medium hot salsa
- 3 tablespoons canola oil
- 2 tablespoons cider vinegar
- 2 large tomatoes, chopped

Combine everything, chill all day, then serve as an appetizer with large taco chips for scooping.

Turkey Balls

- 2 pounds ground turkey breast
- ½ cup dry bread crumbs
- ½ cup milk
- 2 eggs (or egg substitute)
- 1 teaspoon salt
- ½ teaspoon garlic salt

Dump everything in a bowl, moosh around with your hands until thoroughly combined, then form into balls the size of large marbles. Lay out in pans and bake four to five minutes in a 500 oven. Serve in a chafing dish with teriyaki sauce.

Teriyaki Sauce

- 2 tablespoons cornstarch
- ⅓ cup soy sauce
- ¼ cup sugar
- 1 minced clove garlic
- 2 teaspoons minced garlic root
- ¼ cup dry white wine
- 2 cups chicken broth

Blend cornstarch, soy, sugar, garlic and ginger in pan. Stir in wine and broth. Cook, stirring, until it sauce thickens.

Salpicon

- 8 pounds lean top sirloin
- 2 cloves garlic
- 1 bay leaf
- 1 12-ounce can tomatoes
- ¼ cup cilantro leaves
- Salt, pepper
- 1 large bottle zesty Italian dressing
- 1 cup chopped green chilies
- 1 can (about 14 ounces) garbanzo beans
- ½ pound Monterey Jack cheese, cubed
- 2 avocados, in strips
- 1 bunch parsley

If you are planning ahead, look for supermarket specials on thick-cut top sirloin and freeze until you are ready to cook.

When you are ready, plunk the beef hunks into a large pot and cover with water. Add the garlic (smashed), the bay leaf, tomatoes, cilantro and some salt and pepper. Bring to a boil, skim the scum off the top of the pot, then simmer covered about 5 hours.

Let the meat cool, then shred with your hands. Put the shredded meat into a refrigerator container, toss with the salad dressing then cool overnight.

Just before the guests arrive, spread the shredded beef onto a large platter. Top with the garbanzo beans, the chilies, the cubed cheese and strips of avocado. If you want, you can mix a bit of oil and vinegar and spoon lightly over the avocado. Decorate the plate with parsley.

Serve at room temperature. The beef can be served as part of a buffet table (it will feed 20 to 30) or it can be spooned into warm tortillas along with some Mexican salsa.

Clucker Snacks

  2 boneless chicken breasts
  1/3 cup olive oil
  4 cloves garlic, minced
  1/2 teaspoon black pepper
  1/4 teaspoon cayenne pepper
  1/2 cup fine bread crumbs

The breasts should be skinned, boned and cut into bite-sized strips. You should have about one pound.

Marinate the strips in the oil, garlic and black pepper for 30 minutes. Drain.

Mix crumbs with cayenne. Dip strips to coat then arrange on a baking sheet and shove into a 475-degree oven 15 minutes. Remove sheet from oven, turn chicken, sprinkle with salt and cook until browned, probably another five minutes.

Gold Medal Munchies

  1 package round tortilla chips
  2 ripe avocados
  1 teaspoon salt
  2 tablespoons fresh lime juice
  1 medium roma tomato
    Cayenne pepper
  1/3 pound small shrimp

Mash the avocados with a fork and add the salt and lime juice. Chop the tomato into small pieces and add to the avocados. Add cayenne to taste.

I prefer Sesame Blue chips, but you can use any corn tortilla rounds.

Spread the guacamole mixture over the chips and top with three or four tiny shrimp.

It's as easy as that, but this appetizer is best prepared just before eating because the chips can become soggy, in which case the cook may be penalized 4 points in the scoring for lack of artistic merit.

Bed (Time) Spread

  8 ounces nonfat cream cheese
  1 4.5-ounce bottle dried beef
  4 tablespoons skim milk
  2 1/2 teaspoons horseradish

Slice the dried beef and toss into a processor with the other ingredients and blend. Store in a refrigerator crock and, at approximately 11:28 p.m., serve over crackers or hot toast squares. If you want to reduce the salt content, wash the dried beef before slicing it.

Holiday Herb Crackers

  1 pound box oyster crackers
  1 single envelope ranch dressing mix
  1 teaspoon dill weed
  1/2 teaspoon lemon pepper
  1/2 teaspoon garlic salt
  1/2 cup canola oil

Moosh everything around in a large bowl. Spread the crackers over a large cookie pan and shove into a preheated 250-degree oven for 15 minutes. Let cool before you pack them away in an airtight jar or tin.

Sexy Spread

  1 can (15 ounces) garbanzo beans, drained
  2 tablespoons olive oil
  1 tablespoon lemon juice
  2 tablespoons chopped onion
  1 clove garlic, put through press
  1/2 teaspoon salt
  1 teaspoon Worcestershire sauce
  2 tablespoons untoasted sesame seeds
  1/4 teaspoon ground cumin

Put all the ingredients in a blender or food processor until pureed.

Scatter some chopped parsley over the top, if you wish, and serve with hunks of pita bread or with crackers.

Bean Dip '94

  2 tablespoons canola oil
  2/3 cup chopped onion
  1 clove garlic, pureed
  1 1/2 teaspoons ground cumin
  1 teaspoon dried oregano, crumbled
  1/2 teaspoon ground coriander
  1/2 teaspoon chili powder
  1/2 teaspoon salt
  1 can (8 oz.) tomato sauce
  1 can (16 oz.) vegetarian refried beans
    Cayenne pepper

Combine the garlic, salt and spices in a bowl and mix.

In a skillet, cook the onions in the hot oil. When they begin to soften add the ingredients of the bowl and stir-cook for a full minute. Add the tomato sauce and cook another two minutes. Stir in the beans and, when the dip is well mixed, add cayenne pepper to your taste.

Serve at room temperature with taco chips or crackers.

Tapenade Parisian

- 1 cup of Greek olives, pitted
- 2 tablespoons capers
- 1 can (2 ounces) anchovies with oil
- 1 can (6 ounces) firm white tuna
- 2 cloves garlic, peeled
- ½ teaspoon dried thyme
- 1 teaspoon Dijon mustard
- Freshly ground pepper
- ½ teaspoon brandy (optional)
- 1 teaspoon lemon juice
- 4 tablespoons chopped parsley

If you have an ancient cherry pitter (I do), removing the pits from the Greek olives will be simplified. Otherwise, use a small knife to do the job, occasionally uttering a quaint French oath.

What you do is to fling the first eight ingredients into a blender or food processor and create a puree. Remove to a bowl, stir in brandy, lemon juice and parsley and serve with crackers or small slices of baguette.

Olympic Drumroll Drumsticks

- 1¼ cups dry bread crumbs
- 4 teaspoons onion powder
- 4 teaspoons curry powder
- 1½ teaspoons salt
- 1 teaspoon dry mustard
- ½ teaspoon garlic powder
- 1 teaspoon paprika
- ⅛ teaspoon cayenne pepper
- Milk
- 30 chicken drumsticks

Mix together the first eight ingredients. Pour some milk into a bowl.

Grease two cookie sheets and preheat oven to 375 degrees.

Dip each drumstick in milk, then coat in the seasoned crumbs. (Lay out a quarter of the crumbs on a sheet of waxed paper. Then add more crumbs as needed. If you lay out all the crumbs at once, they'll soak up milk, form into little balls and, well, I can't even bear to think about it!)

Lay the coated drumsticks out on the cookie sheets and bake in the oven for 45 minutes to one hour, or until the crumbs are a dark golden brown.

The host might want to finish cooking about 60 to 90 minutes before the guests arrive so the drumsticks will be at room temperature. They lose some of their pizazz when refrigerated.

Baked Clams

- 1 onion, minced
- 1 clove garlic, minced
- 1 can (6 ounces) minced clams
- 1 cup bread crumbs
- 1 tablespoon lemon juice
- 2 tablespoons white wine
- ¼ cup grated Parmesan cheese
- 1 tablespoon chopped parsley
- 1 teaspoon dried oregano
- Salt, pepper
- Olive oil

In a small skillet, heat some oil and add the onion and garlic. When the onion begins to relax, dump in the clams (including their liquid), bread crumbs, lemon juice, wine, cheese, parsley and oregano, and salt and pepper to taste. (It may not need any.)

Stuff this mess into clam shells. Shove the stuffed shells into a 350-degree oven for 10 minutes.

Prawn Appetizer

- 2 pounds prawns
- 1 lemon, thinly sliced
- 1 red onion, peeled and thinly sliced
- 1 cup pitted black olives
- ¼ cup olive oil
- 2 cloves garlic, mashed
- 1 tablespoon dry mustard
- ½ tablespoon salt
- ½ cup lemon juice
- 1 tablespoon red wine vinegar
- dash of cayenne pepper

Peel the prawns and drop into boiling salted water for 90 seconds. Remove and save in cold water.

Drain, pat dry and dump into a serving bowl. Mix all the other ingredients, pour over the prawns and let refrigerate for two hours. Remove from the cooler when your guests arrive and serve with toothpicks, to stab the little critters.

Antipasto Spread

- 1 can (4 ounces) sardines
- 1 can anchovy fillets
- 1 teaspoon lemon juice
- 6 ounces non-fat cream cheese
- 1 tablespoon cognac

Sardines are another rediscovered wonder food and taste a whole lot better than the cod liver oil which was inflicted upon offspring by an earlier generation of mothers.

For this spread simply mix all the ingredients in a blender and serve at room temperature with crackers or toast rounds.

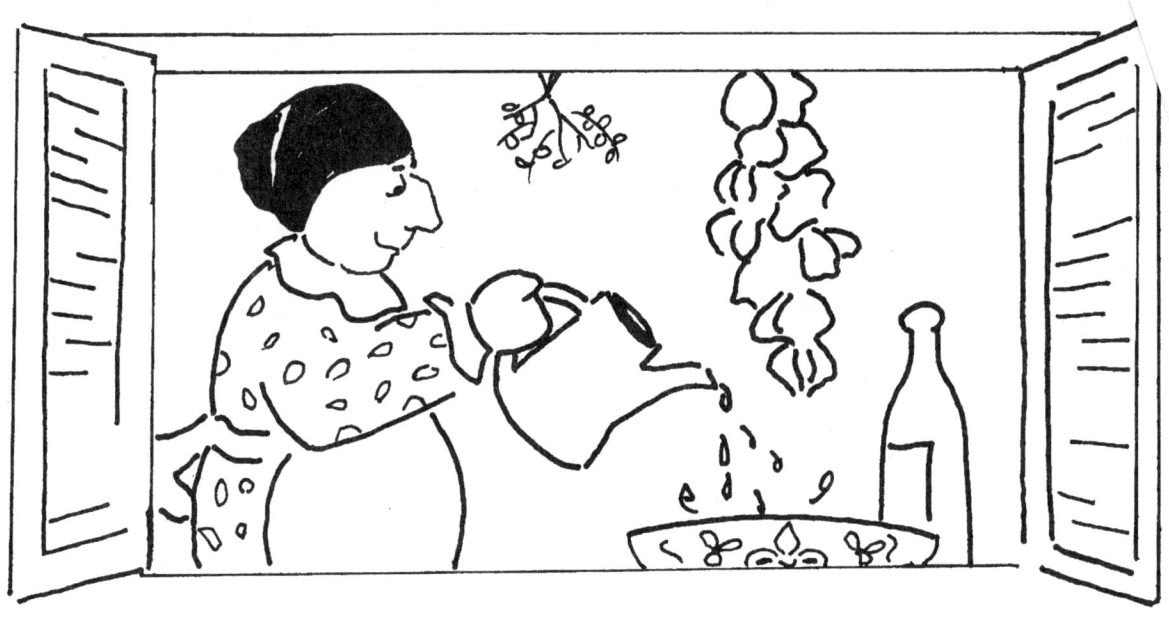

ITALIAN PASTA AND ASIAN NOODLES

Do all the residents of Sicily live to be 105? Or do all the residents of Sicily look to be 105 when they're actually celebrating their 38th birthdays?

The Intermediate Eater has been wrestling with questions like those as a part of continuing research into diet, health and long life. Studies conducted in this country and abroad indicate the Italians are particularly robust and thus warrant close scrutiny.

If you've ever been to Rome you know that Italians wave their arms a whole lot. Perhaps it improves their circulation. They also like to yell, frequently and at full pitch, usually at major traffic intersections. Is it a coincidence they are blessed with strong lungs, as exhibited by operatic tenors like Caruso, Lanza, Pavarotti and a thousand shower-stall imitators?

The Intermediate Eater has his own pet theory. Ergo, Italians multiply and thrive for three reasons: Garlic, olive oil and good wine.

Scientific studies indicate that wine and garlic lower levels of "bad" cholesterol in the blood. Additional and recent research, reported by health and diet expert Dr. Kenneth Cooper, suggests that an olive oil-rich diet is even healthier than the so-called low-fat regimens.

It doesn't work with every oil, mind you. Olive and canola oils seem to have this particular attribute.

I stood outside a cafe kitchen in Venice one afternoon, peering at the cooks over the herb-filled pots lined up on an open window. The women sauteed virtually every dish in copious amounts of olive oil. Then, before dishing up the entree, they coated the bottom of the serving platter with another small lake of olive oil.

Of course everybody in the joint looked like an offensive guard for the Green Bay Packers. But the cooks and customers all wore extremely contented expressions, as though they alone knew the three secrets to the good life.

Olive oil, garlic and good wine.

Locally, we have noted that the food servers at many Italian restaurants now bring customers cut slices of chewy bread and – instead of butter – a saucer of olive oil for dipping.

You might extend your own research with dishes like those in this chapter.

Happy Holiday Lasagne

- 1 whole chicken
- 1 onion
- Handful of celery tops
- ¼ cup olive oil
- 1 chicken bouillon cube
- ½ cup flour
- ½ teaspoon salt
- ½ teaspoon dry basil
- 1/8 teaspoon nutmeg
- 2 cups (1 pound) creamed cottage cheese
- 1 egg, slightly beaten
- ½ pound lasagne noodles, cooked and drained
- 1 package frozen chopped spinach, thawed and squeeze dried
- ¼ pound sliced mozzarella cheese
- ½ cup grated Parmesan cheese
- 1/3 cup peeled red pepper cut in strips

Toss the bird in a pot, add salted water to cover and toss in the onion, quartered, and the celery tops. Simmer until done, then let cool. Meanwhile let the spinach thaw, then squeeze it dry.

When the chicken is cool, remove skin and bones, saving the broth. Dice the chicken meat. You'll need 2 ½ cups for this recipe and if there is extra, you can save it for a sandwich or two tomorrow.

OK, heat the olive oil in a saucepan. Blend in the flour, salt and basil.

When you have a smooth paste, slowly stir in 3 cups of the reserved chicken broth. Add the bouillon cube, too. Stir-cook until the sauce thickens. Remove from heat and add the chicken meat and nutmeg, freshly grated if possible.

Mix the cottage cheese with the beaten egg.

Lightly grease a 9-by-13-inch oven dish. Place a third of the chicken mixture on the bottom, top with half the noodles, half the cottage cheese mixture, half the spinach and half the mozzarella. Repeat layers then top with the final third of the chicken mixture and the Parmesan. Lay the strips of peeled red pepper over the top. (You can find them in jars at any supermarket.)

Bake the lasagne 45 minutes in a 375-degree oven. Remove and let stand 10 minutes before cutting into 6 portions.

Maestro's Manicotti

Filling:

- ¾ pound Dungeness crab meat
- ½ pound small Oregon shrimp
- 4 diced green onions, including green tops
- 1 cup (4 ounces) grated fontina cheese
- 16 dry manicotti shells
- ½ cup freshly grated Romano cheese

Cook the manicotti shells in salted, boiling water to instructions on the package. (I used Ronzoni large manicotti shells. Cook a couple of extra shells in case one or more breaks up in the cooking.) Drain the shells on paper towels.

Mix together the crab, shrimp, onions and the fontina. With your fingers, stuff the crab mixture into the shells. (Scandinavian fontina cheese is probably cheaper in your market than the Italian variety. For this dish, you probably won't notice any difference.) No, I didn't forget the Romano cheese.

It will be added to the dish later.

Red Sauce:

- 2 tablespoons olive oil
- 1 onion, diced
- 1 carrot, peeled and grated
- 1 can (1 pound) smashed tomatoes
- 1 cup chicken broth
- 1 teaspoon basil

Heat the oil in a saucepan. Saute the onion and carrot about three minutes.

Add tomatoes with their liquid, plus the chicken broth and basil. Simmer this mess for about 30 minutes.

White Sauce:

- 1/3 cup olive oil (or butter if you prefer)
- 1 small onion, minced
- 4 tablespoons flour
- 1/8 teaspoon grated nutmeg
- ¾ cup milk
- ¾ cup chicken broth
- 1 cup (4 ounces) grated fontina cheese

Heat the olive oil in a skillet and saute the onion three minutes. Stir in the flour and nutmeg. When you have a smooth sludge, slowly add the broth and milk. Stir-cook until you have a medium white sauce, then stir in the cheese. If the sauce is too thick, you still can add more broth at this point.

To build this masterpiece, grease one large or two medium-sized Pyrex oven dishes. Spread the red sauce over the bottom. Top with the filled manicotti shells. Pour the white sauce over the top and sprinkle with the half-cup of grated Romano cheese.

Shove the dishes into a preheated 400-degree oven for about 30 minutes. Let rest for 3-5 minutes after you remove from the oven, then serve to eight guests along with Italian or French bread and maybe a side dish of cooked green beans.

Emerald City Manicotti

  8 to 10 manicotti shells
    2 tablespoons olive oil or butter
    3 tablespoons green onions
  10 ounces frozen spinach
    1 cup cooked chicken
    1 cup ham
    ½ cup Romano cheese
    2 eggs, beaten
    1 teaspoon Italian seasoning
    ¼ teaspoon freshly ground pepper
      Romano sauce (recipe follows)

Mince the green onion, chicken and ham into small pieces. Thaw the spinach and squeeze dry in your fist. Grate the cheese.

OK, now you should melt the butter in a large skillet and saute the green onions for a couple of minutes. Remove the pan from the heat and add the spinach, chicken, ham, cheese, the seasonings and the beaten eggs. Mix everything.

Next, heat water to boiling in a large pot, add salt and toss in the manicotti shells. Cook 8 minutes (or according to package instructions). Drain the pasta, then add cold water to the pot.

Remove the manicotti shells one by one, shake off the excess water and, using your fingers, stuff them with the ham-chicken mixture.

Grease an oven dish large enough to hold all the pasta tubes. Lay out the stuffed manicotti and, if you have any filling left, scatter over top.

Pour the Romano sauce over the filled tubes, then shove the dish into a preheated, 350-degree oven for 20 minutes. Turn the oven heat to broil and partially brown the sauce on top for a minute or two.

Romano Sauce:

    ¼ cup olive oil or butter
    1 clove garlic, mashed
    ¼ cup flour
    2 teaspoons chicken bouillon powder
    2 cups half and half
    1 cup grated Romano cheese

Saute the garlic in the butter for a minute. Stir in the flour and chicken bouillon and stir-cook until smooth. Remove the skillet from the heat and add the half and half.

Return to the heat and bring to a simmer, stirring. When the sauce has thickened, remove from the heat again and stir in the cheese.

You can use egg substitute like Second Nature in the stuffing and whole milk instead of half and half in the sauce.

This should serve four to five.

Puffin Pasta

    1 pound pennine pasta
    ¼ cup olive oil
    4 cloves garlic, minced
    2 tablespoons anchovy paste
    4 cups cooked broccoli florets
      Fresh pepper

Cook and drain the pennine, which is small tube (or penne) pasta. You can use any similar pasta but it doesn't work very well with long strands of spaghetti or fettuccine.

While the pasta is cooking in the boiling, salted water, heat the oil in a skillet. Add the garlic and cook carefully, to make sure it doesn't turn brown and bitter. Stir in the anchovy paste.

Drain the pasta and dump it into the skillet. Add the broccoli and toss carefully but thoroughly. Top with lots of freshly grated pepper.

A meal like this supplies enough carbohydrates to fuel one healthful walk, four rounds of golf or 32 bird-watching expeditions.

Green Olive Pesto

    1 firmly packed cup of green olives with pimentos
    ⅓ cup walnuts
    1 clove garlic, minced
    1 cup parsley leaves
    ¼ cup olive oil
    2 tablespoons parmesan cheese
      Salt, if needed

Pat the olives dry with a paper towel, then toss into a processor with the nuts, garlic and parsley. With the machine running slowly add the oil in a drizzle. Then blend in the parmesan, and be sure it is freshly grated. Add salt to taste.

You can use this green gloop as an appetizer dip. Or if you are serving it atop something like Italian penne, save some of the pasta water to thin the pesto. Then toss it repeatedly with the drained but still hot pasta.

Leftover pesto will keep a few weeks in the refrigerator, if you cover the top of the container with olive oil.

Homerun Noodles

  1 pound spaghetti or fettuccine
1½ cups broccoli florets
1½ cups snow peas
  1 sweet red pepper, cut in strips
  1 cup carrot, in matchstick slices
10 large mushrooms
  2 tablespoons olive oil
  2 cloves garlic, minced
  ¼ cup minced parsley
  ¼ cup chopped fresh basil (or 1 teaspoon dried)
    Salt and pepper
  ¼ cup grated Parmesan cheese
  1 cup sour cream
  2 cups cooked chicken, in thin strips (optional)

Bring a pan of water to a slow boil and toss in the broccoli, sweet pepper and carrot sticks. After 30 seconds add the pea pods and cook another 30 seconds (1 minute total for the veggies, no more). Drain and reserve.

While the pasta is cooking in boiling salted water, heat the oil in a skillet and add the minced garlic, parsley and sliced mushrooms. Also add the cooked chicken at this point, if you choose. Season with salt, pepper and basil. Add the Parmesan cheese, sour cream and mix with a spoon.

Quickly drain the pasta and plunk into a warm dish. Add the mushroom mixture, the parboiled veggies, toss quickly and serve. This is sufficient for four to six portions, depending upon whatever else you plan to serve the hungry horde.

Pender Street Noodles

  2 whole chicken breasts
  1 pound spaghetti
⅓ cup peanut butter
  2 tablespoons white wine vinegar
  ½ tablespoon soy sauce
  2 teaspoons sugar
  2 teaspoons canola oil
  1 teaspoon sesame oil
  2 green onions with tops, chopped
  ½ teaspoon dried red pepper flakes
⅔ cup plain yogurt
  1 1-inch hunk fresh ginger root, peeled
  1 clove garlic, peeled
  ½ teaspoon salt
  2 carrots, peeled and cut in thin strips
  1 red bell pepper cut in thin strips
  ½ cup chopped fresh cilantro leaves

This recipe was inspired by a trip to Vancouver, so while humming "Oh, Canada," cut the chicken breasts in two and poach or cook in microwave just until no longer red in the middle. Cut chicken meat diagonally into strips.

Cook the spaghetti in boiling salted water until done. Drain, spread out on a cookie sheet and cool in the refrigerator.

Plunk the peanut butter, vinegar, soy sauce, sugar, canola oil, sesame oil, green onions, pepper flakes, yogurt, ginger root, garlic and salt into a food processor or blender. Puree into a sludge.

Toss the cooled noodles with the sauce, carrot strips, pepper strips and half the chicken strips. Top with the remaining chicken strips and the cilantro. Serves six, chilled or at room temperature.

Peanut Pasta

    Pasta to serve 2 people
  2 cups broccoli florets
⅓ cup peanut butter
  ½ cup hot chicken broth
  1 teaspoon soy sauce
  2 tablespoons rice vinegar
  2 tablespoons canola oil
  2 cloves minced garlic
  1 teaspoon crushed red pepper flakes, or to taste

I prefer to use small pasta shells or tubes like penne. Cook in boiling, salted water until tender to the bite. Steam the broccoli florets 3 minutes.

Meanwhile heat the canola oil in a saucepan and saute the garlic for a minute over medium low heat. Add the peanut butter, hot chicken broth, soy sauce, vinegar and hot pepper flakes to taste. Stir until smooth and remove from heat.

Serve the pasta up on two plates, top with the sauce and toss on the hot broccoli.

McPasta

  ¼ pound smoked salmon
  1 cup cream (or low-fat evaporated milk)
  1 tablespoon green onion, chopped
  2 tablespoons white wine
    Salt, pepper
  1 cup frozen peas, thawed
    Penne pasta to serve two, cooked

Put half the salmon into a blender along with 2 tablespoons of cream and the green onion. Lean on the button until you have a puree.

Heat the wine in a skillet, add the rest of the cream and the salmon puree and simmer (don't boil) until it is hot and thick. Add salt and pepper if needed. Stir in the peas and let heat for a minute.

When the penne is done, drain quickly and dump it into the skillet. Stir once or twice then serve up into 2 large bowls, scattering over the top the rest of the smoked salmon, crumbled.

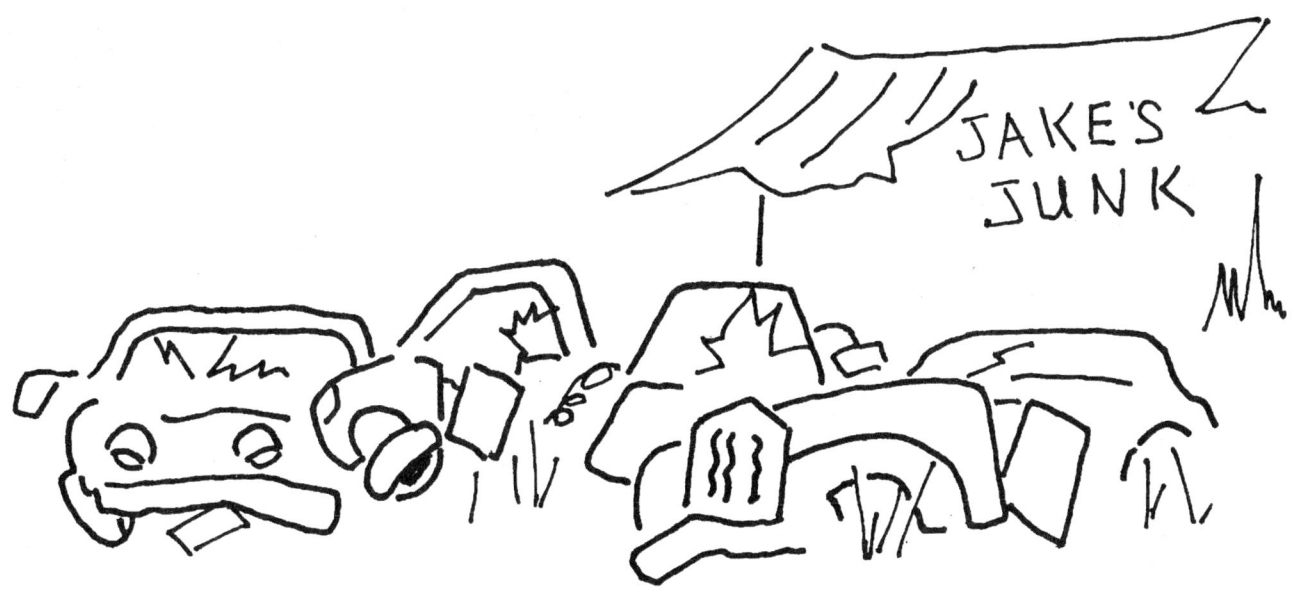

POULTRY

What year were you born? Check out the used car lots and see if you can spot a Plymouth, Ford, Studebaker or Hudson built the same year. Despite the fact that it was operated no more than two hours a day, on average, it is today a bucket of bolts. Meanwhile you are still humming along through 18-hour days, accelerating up hills, around blind curves, pausing only infrequently to refuel on a cup of coffee and two sugar doughnuts.

The Human Machine is a wonder to behold. Consider the miracles the body daily performs without the aid of batteries, computer chips or frequent front-end alignments.

If you are the typical American, you now spend approximately 16 seconds each morning gulping down your daily allotment of vitamins. In the evening you might take an aspirin or two. Your apple a day is supposed to keep the doctor away and a forkful or two of broccoli might also postpone your next date with a nurse.

Some vitamins do wonders for the larynx and esophagus. Others preserve or enhance the eyesight. Vitamin E seems to strengthen the heart. Vitamin C may reduce the sniffles.

As for the aspirin, it seems to work equally well on headaches, tennis elbow and throbbing wisdom teeth.

One recent morning, Yr. Obdt. Correspondent popped five pills in rapid succession. There was an aspirin to thin the blood, a vitamin C tablet, a vitamin E capsule, a multivitamin scatterpill and a mysterious little red pebble prescribed by my doctor to eliminate some fungus on my big toenail.

How does the body separate the various vitamins and dispatch them to the nose, liver, larynx and duodenum without missing or mixing? When does the aspirin learn that my elbow, head and teeth are pain free but that I can use a little help thinning the blood? And how does that little red pill know it is supposed to proceed directly from the gullet to my big toe?

It's a mystery and poses a lot of questions I ponder while munching on a chicken leg or some other health foods like those in this chapter.

Drumstick Dinner

- 4 turkey drumsticks
- ¼ cup olive oil
- 1 clove garlic, minced
- 1 large onion, sliced
- 1½ cups chopped carrots
- 1½ cups sliced celery
- ½ cup chicken broth
- ½ cup white wine
- 1 teaspoon seasoned salt
- ⅛ teaspoon pepper
- 1 tablespoon flour

Brown the legs in the hot olive oil. Add the garlic, onion, celery and carrots. Saute until the onions begin to relax, then add the broth, wine, seasoned salt and pepper. Bring to a boil, reduce heat and simmer two hours.

Remove turkey and vegetables with a slotted spoon. Stir the flour into some of the liquid from the pan to make a paste. Stir this back in and boil the sauce to thicken.

Return the turkey and veggies to the pan and when hot serve up on a big platter.

If you like white meat, substitute a pound and a half of turkey tenders for the drumsticks. Just cut them into hunks and you probably won't have to braise the dish quite as long.

Cadillac Chicken

- 1 package "best of chicken"
- ⅔ cup buttermilk
- ⅓ cup lemon juice
- Olive oil
- 12 chopped sage leaves (or 1 teaspoon powdered)
- 2 teaspoons salt
- 1 teaspoon cayenne pepper
- ¾ cup yellow cornmeal
- ½ cup dry bread crumbs
- ¼ cup grated Parmesan cheese
- ¼ cup minced parsley
- ½ teaspoon paprika
- 2 eggs

The best-of-chicken packages should include two chicken breast halves, two drumstick-and-thigh portions and two wings. I usually remove excess skin or fat but I leave the skin on the wings and drumstick portions. First, though, cut off wing tips and whack the remaining portion in half at the joint.

This gives you a breast serving for two guests, thigh-drumstick portions for two guests and one wing portion for everybody.

In the morning, mix together the buttermilk, lemon juice, olive oil, the sage, one teaspoon salt and a half teaspoon of cayenne. Put the chicken pieces in a plastic refrigerator dish, pour the buttermilk muck over the top and let sit refrigerated all day, turning the chicken a couple of times.

Near dinnertime combine on a plate or piece of waxed paper the cornmeal, bread crumbs, Parmesan, parsley, paprika, the other teaspoon of salt and the final half teaspoon of cayenne.

In a bowl beat the eggs with two tablespoons cold water.

Remove chicken from the refrigerator. Lift each piece from the buttermilk swamp, dip in the egg wash, then roll to cover in that cornmeal mess. All parts of each piece should be covered.

Then carefully lay the chicken out on a rack and let sit for 30 to 45 minutes.

Preheat oven to 425 degrees. Lightly grease a cookie pan. Lay out the chicken pieces. Moisten the top of each piece with a bit more olive oil (or you can use melted butter if you prefer).

Shove the pan into the oven, and the chicken should be perfectly cooked in 30 to 35 minutes.

With mashed potatoes and mixed veggies, this will serve four auto mechanics after they've washed their hands and faces.

The Lemon Chicken Caper

- 4 skinned and boned chicken breasts (8 pieces)
- Salt
- Pepper
- ½ teaspoon powdered sage
- ¾ cup flour
- 4 tablespoons olive oil
- 3 garlic cloves, minced
- 1½ pounds fresh mushrooms
- 4 teaspoons lemon juice
- ¾ cup dry white wine
- 1 tablespoon capers

Pound the breast portions to flatten slightly. Mix the salt, pepper and sage with the flour and lightly dredge the chicken.

Heat the oil in a large skillet. Brown the chicken on both sides, just until golden. Remove to a warm dish. Add the sliced mushrooms to the pan along with the garlic. When the mushrooms no longer look like toadstools, add the lemon juice and wine. Return the chicken pieces to the pan, cover the skillet and simmer until the breasts are cooked, about 15 minutes.

Add the capers, stir around for a minute, then serve to six or eight guests with the mushrooms and pan liquid over the top.

Portuguese Chicken

- 1 best of fryer, cut up
- olive oil
- Salt, pepper
- 4 ounces ham, cubed
- 1 small onion, chopped
- 1 tablespoon flour
- 3 tablespoons parsley, chopped
- 1 cup chicken broth
- 2 large cloves garlic
- 12 hazelnuts

In a skillet or stove-top casserole heat some olive oil and brown the chicken on all sides, sprinkling with salt and pepper. Remove chicken. Add to the pan the ham and onion, saute 3 minutes. Stir in flour and stir-cook another minute. Add the chicken broth to the pan, stir-cook to thicken, then pour this sludge over the chicken when you return the clucker pieces to the pan.

Bring liquid to a slow boil and simmer for 40 minutes.

Toast the hazelnuts, then grind in a mortar with the garlic and parsley.

After the chicken has cooked 40 minutes, stir in the hazelnut mixture and cook another 5 minutes.

Serve with noodles or mashed potatoes.

Kauai Chicken

- 1 best of fryer
- 6 cloves garlic, pureed
- 3 slices ginger root
- 2 green onions, chopped
- 2 tablespoons honey
- ½ teaspoon black pepper
- 2½ tablespoons Oriental fish sauce
- 1 teaspoon sesame oil
- 1 tablespoon canola oil
- 1 tablespoon sherry
- 1 teaspoon orange zest
- ⅔ cups orange juice

Cut the fryer into serving pieces. Remove skin from breast and thighs if you desire.

Dump the pureed garlic into a bowl. Add the ginger slices and green onion.

With a blunt instrument smash the ginger and onion until it is incorporated into the garlic. Add the other ingredients to the bowl.

Place the chicken pieces in a refrigerator dish. Top with the garlic muck, stir everything around with a Polynesian back scratcher, cover and let sit refrigerated overnight or all day.

Forty minutes before dinner, plunk the chicken pieces on a cookie sheet and shove into an oven preheated to 450 degrees. After 20 minutes remove from oven, baste with the marinade and return to oven for a final 15 minutes, or until brown and crisp.

Walnut Sauce for Chicken

- 1 cup walnuts
- 1 large clove garlic
- 1½ teaspoons dried coriander
- 1 teaspoon paprika
- Dash of cayenne
- 2 teaspoons white wine vinegar
- 1 cup chicken broth
- Salt to taste

Dump walnuts and peeled clove of garlic into a blender or food processor.

Hit the button and add just a tablespoon or two of water, slowly, until you have a paste. Remove to a bowl and add the coriander, paprika and cayenne. Add the broth, slowly while stirring, because you'll just need enough to create a sauce the consistency of thick cream. Add the vinegar and salt to taste.

This is enough sauce to accompany six broiled chicken breasts. Spread the sauce over one portion of the plate and top with the chicken.

Artichoke Chicken

- 6 half chicken breasts
- 2 tablespoons olive oil
- ½ pound fresh mushrooms, sliced
- 3 cloves garlic, minced
- 2 tablespoons capers
- 1 can artichoke hearts (about six) halved
- 1 cup dry white wine
- ½ cup fresh, diced tomatoes
- 1 lemon
- ¼ cup green onions, chopped

Heat oil in skillet and lightly brown chicken on both sides. Remove to a warm oven. Dump the mushrooms, garlic, capers and artichoke hearts into the pan. Stir around, then add the wine and stir again. Add the tomatoes, the juice from the lemon and the green onions. Stir until sauce thickens and reduces. Return chicken to the pan and serve when it is warmed through. Feeds six with pasta or rice.

Put That Down or I'll Break Your Wrist!

(Grams of unhealthy trans fat in the following packaged foods)

Pound Cake	4.5
Doughnuts	4.0
Frozen French Fries	3.0
Snack Crackers	2.5
Taco Shells	2.5

Chicken Vesuvio

- 1 fryer, cut up
- ⅓ cup flour
- 1½ teaspoons dried basil
- ¾ teaspoon dried oregano
- ¾ teaspoon dried sage
- ½ teaspoon salt
- ¼ teaspoon freshly ground pepper
- ½ cup olive oil
- 3 baking potatoes
- 3 cloves minced garlic
- ¾ cup dry white wine
- ⅓ cup minced parsley

Rinse and dry chicken parts. Mix together flour, salt, pepper and herbs and dredge chicken in this mess.

Heat oil in a large skillet. Add chicken in one layer, fry until golden brown on both sides, about 15 minutes. Remove chicken to a large oven dish.

Cut washed potatoes lengthwise into wedges. Fry in the oil remaining in skillet, until lightly brown on all sides. Remove to the oven dish with the chicken. Remove all but two tablespoons oil from skillet. Add wine, mix with pan juices then pour all this sludge over the chicken and potatoes. Sprinkle with garlic and parsley, then shove the dish into a 375-degree oven. Cook 20 to 25 minutes, then let stand five minutes before serving to four famished fans.

In baseball announcer Harry Caray's recipe, served at his Chicago restaurant, thawed peas are added to the casserole with the browned chicken and potatoes.

Skaters' Thighs

- 5 pounds boned and skinned chicken thighs
- 2 tablespoons sesame oil
- ½ teaspoon Tabasco sauce
- 2 cloves garlic, minced
- 2 pieces ginger root, crushed
- ¼ cup chopped onion
- ⅓ cup sugar
- ½ cup soy sauce
- 4 tablespoons white wine
- Sesame seeds

Marinate the thighs in the sauce constructed from the next eight ingredients for an hour. Broil chicken on both sides until done. Sprinkle liberally with sesame seeds and this should serve 10 guests as an entree with rice. (However you may have to crack a few guests over the knuckles with a wooden spoon if they neglect to leave a few thighs for your late-night snacking.)

Chicken and Mushrooms

- 4 large chicken thighs
- ⅓ cup sun-dried tomatoes
- 1 small onion, minced
- 2 cloves garlic, minced
- ½ teaspoon dried basil
- ¼ teaspoon red pepper flakes
- ½ pound mushrooms, thick sliced
- ½ cup dry white wine
- ½ cup chicken broth
- 2 tablespoons tomato ketchup

Sun-dried tomatoes are marketed either dry, in envelopes, or oil-packed, in jars. If you are using the dry version, cut in thin strips and soak in oil for awhile. Then add to the skillet with the wine and broth. If you are using tomatoes already packed in oil, cut in strips and add during the last two minutes of the total cooking process.

In either event, pour into a skillet two tablespoons of the oil in which the tomatoes have been soaking. When the oil is hot, salt and pepper the chicken thighs (I prefer them skinned) and brown them on both sides in the pan.

Remove the thighs to a warm plate. Reduce heat under the pan and add the onions, garlic, basil and red pepper flakes. Saute about two minutes, stirring, then add the mushrooms and cook another four minutes. Next add the wine, broth and the ketchup. Bring the liquid to a boil, return the chicken to the pan and simmer 15 minutes, covered.

Uncover the pan and continue to simmer the ingredients until the liquids have been reduced and thickened.

This will serve two and I prefer it accompanied by penne pasta, cooked al dente and then tossed with olive oil and a bit of parmesan cheese.

Apricot Chicken

- 1 cut up chicken, or equivalent
- Poultry seasoning
- 1 cup apricot preserves
- 1 packet onion soup mix
- ¼ cup lemon juice
- 4 tablespoons Worcestershire sauce

Season chicken with poultry seasoning and place in baking pan. Bake 40 minutes at 350 degrees. Meanwhile, mix preserves with onion soup mix, lemon and Worcestershire.

Pour over chicken and bake another 20 minutes. Put under broiler to crisp, if desired. Serve with oven-browned potatoes and, oh, maybe a boiled cabbage like they serve in London, WC2H9OJ, England.

Hawaiian Chicken

    3 chicken breasts, boned and halved
    2 eggs, slightly beaten
    2 cups dry bread crumbs
    ½ teaspoon each salt, thyme and paprika
    2 tablespoons olive oil or butter
    2 cups pineapple juice
    2 tablespoons lemon juice
    2 tablespoons cornstarch
    1 teaspoon curry powder
    1 teaspoon powdered ginger
    2 tablespoons sugar
    ½ cup macadamia nuts, coarsely chopped

Mix the crumbs with the salt, thyme and paprika. Dip chicken breasts (with or without the skin) in the eggs, then in the seasoned crumbs.

Heat the oil or butter in a large skillet and saute the chicken until golden brown on both sides. Remove to a platter and set aside.

In the same skillet combine the pineapple juice, lemon juice, cornstarch, curry, ginger and sugar. Moosh this around with a wooden spoon then return the chicken to the pan and slop some sauce over each portion. Cover the skillet and simmer the ingredients 20 to 30 minutes, or until tender.

Remove chicken to the platter again, pour the sauce over the top and finish with a scattering of nuts.

With rice, this will serve six mainlanders, four Hawaiians or one Samoan.

Open-Faced Option

    1 medium onion, minced
    1 clove garlic, minced
    2 teaspoons chili powder
    ½ teaspoon ground cumin
    1 tablespoon canola oil
    1 pound lean ground turkey or beef
    1 can (8 ounces) tomato sauce
    ½ cup bottled barbecue sauce
    1 can (4 ounces) diced green chilies
    1 can (3 ounces) sliced ripe olives, drained

You have the option of using ground turkey or low-fat ground beef in this recipe.

Heat the oil in a pot. Add the onion and garlic and sprinkle with the chili powder and cumin. After 2 minutes stir in the turkey or beef and cook about 4 minutes, busting up the meat with a wooden spoon.

Moosh in the rest of the ingredients and again you can exercise your option. Use mild chilies, jalapenos or a combination of the two. Simmer the resultant mess for about 5 minutes then serve over toast or toasted hamburger buns. This will make four or more open-faced sandwiches. You have the further option of sharing them with your friends. or eating them all yourself.

Like Chocolate for Chicken

    2 tablespoons sesame seeds
    3 tablespoon canola oil
    8 medium chicken thighs
       Salt, pepper
    1½ cups chopped onion
    2 cloves garlic, minced
    1½ tablespoons chili powder
    ½ teaspoon cinnamon
    ½ teaspoon coriander
    24 ounces canned tomatoes, with juices
    ¾ cup chicken broth
    1½ teaspoons sugar
    1 ounce unsweetened chocolate, chopped

Toast the sesame seeds in a skillet in the oven, but take care you don't incinerate them.

Heat the oil in a skillet. Salt and pepper the chicken, saute over medium heat about 10 minutes, then remove from the pan. Pour off all but two tablespoons pan drippings. Add the onion and cook a minute. Dump in the garlic and spices and cook another minute. Add the tomatoes, breaking up with a spoon. Then stir in the broth, sugar and chocolate. Return the chicken to the pan and simmer, partly covered, for 10 or 15 minutes until done.

Sprinkle the sesame seeds over the top of the chicken. It should serve four with cooked rice or noodles and an avocado salad.

Norma's Chicken

    4 whole boneless, skinned chicken breasts
    8 ounces low-fat Swiss cheese
    1 can undiluted cream of celery soup
    ¼ cup dry white wine
    2 cups packaged poultry dressing
    ⅓ cup melted butter
       Pepper to taste

Cut the breasts in half to give you eight pieces. Lay out snugly in an oven dish to fit. Top the breasts with slices of the cheese. Mix the dry, packaged dressing with the butter. (Crumble the dressing first, if you are using croutons.) Sprinkle this mess over the cheese.

Mix the soup and wine, pour this slop over the top and bake the chicken uncovered, 50 to 60 minutes at 350 degrees.

It serves eight, and Norma Bruns says you can substitute cream of chicken or mushroom soup, but she prefers the celery. So there!

Pollo Extra-Olive

    1/3 cup olive oil
     1   small onion, chopped
     2   cloves garlic, minced
     ½   cup dry white wine
     2   cups canned roma tomatoes, seeded and chopped
    12   large black pitted olives, quartered
         Salt, pepper to taste
     4   chicken breast pieces
    12   fresh basil leaves, shredded

You want to include the juices with the tomatoes and don't have a cow if you let a few seeds slip into the sauce.

If you don't have or don't want to fork out for the fresh basil leaves you could substitute chopped parsley. But it won't be quite the same, Rosa.

Slightly flatten the chicken (2 whole breasts divided into 4 pieces) by placing between pieces of waxed paper and whacking with a blunt object, the approximate size and heft of a Rome traffic cop's billy club.

Heat half the oil in a skillet. Add the onion and saute 4 minutes, or until it has softened. Add the garlic and cook another minute. Dump in the wine and boil down by half. Add the tomatoes and olives and simmer for 5 minutes. Salt and pepper to taste.

In another large skillet heat the rest of the oil. Saute the chicken breasts until golden on both sides. Don't overcook.

Dump the tomato sauce atop the breasts and simmer over low heat for a minute or so. Remove the breasts to four warm plates. To the sauce left in the pan add the basil, stir-cook 20 seconds, then spoon over the breasts.

10-Minute Turkey Dinner (Sauteed turkey breasts)

     1   pound raw, turkey breast cutlets
         Salt, pepper
     3   tablespoons butter
    1/3 cup sliced almonds
     3   tablespoons minced green onions
     ¼   cup white wine
     ½   cup chicken stock

Salt and pepper the cutlets, then saute three minutes per side in a skillet containing the melted butter. Remove turkey to a warm dish. Add almonds to the pan and saute until golden. Remove them, too.

Saute the onion in remaining pan liquids. Raise heat, add wine and broth and cook down two minutes. Spoon the sauce over the turkey slices and sprinkle with the almonds.

You could serve this to four guests with some noodles cooked, drained and tossed with a bit of Dijon mustard.

Far East Chicken

     2   chicken breasts
     6   green onions
     3   tablespoons soy sauce
     1   teaspoon sesame oil
     1   tablespoon sherry
     1   teaspoon salt
     5   tablespoons peanut oil
     2   tablespoons chopped ginger root
     2   tablespoons chopped garlic cloves
     2   tablespoons Hoisin sauce

Skin and bone the chicken then cut into 1 ½-inch chunks. Cut the onions, including most of the green tops, in ½-inch sections.

Moosh together the chicken, onions, soy sauce, sesame oil, sherry and salt. Let sit for an hour or so.

When you are ready to cook, heat the peanut oil in a skillet or wok, medium high. Toss in the ginger and garlic and stir-cook 15 seconds. Add the Hoisin sauce. Add a tablespoon of water to that chicken mess in the other bowl and dump all this into the pan, too. Stir-cook until the chicken is done. Then serve over rice.

Jean Burgan says this recipe serves two, but you have to take into consideration the fact that her husband is a charter member of The Clean Plate Club.

The Gopher's Game Hens

    1/3 cup Dijon mustard
     2   minced green onions
     ¼   cup fresh lime juice
     2   teaspoons honey
         Pepper
     4   tablespoons butter, melted
     2   game hens

Split hens and marinate in a mixture of the remaining ingredients for at least an hour.

Broil hens 5 minutes on each side, turn heat to 450 degrees and cook another 30 minutes or until done, basting.

I can eat a whole game hen myself, but for more modest appetites this may serve four, with a wild-rice mixture and salad on the side.

Leavenworth Chicken

- 8 large chicken thighs
- ½ teaspoon salt
- ¼ teaspoon garlic salt
- ½ teaspoon onion powder
- ½ teaspoon black pepper
- ½ teaspoon oregano
- 2 tablespoons olive oil
- 1 large onion, chopped
- 2 cloves garlic, minced or mashed
- ¼ cup paprika
- 1 can (6 ounces) tomato paste
- 2½ cups chicken broth
- 8 ounces sour cream
- Cooked noodles to serve 4

Mix together the salt, garlic salt, onion powder, pepper and oregano. Rub this into the chicken thighs (I prefer to skin them first). Then brown the chicken, turning in hot oil.

Remove the chicken from the pan and keep warm. Into the same skillet dump the onions. Cook 2 minutes over medium heat, then add the garlic and paprika.

Cook another minute, then stir in the tomato paste and broth.

Simmer 30 seconds, then return the chicken to the sauce in the pan, cover and simmer 25 minutes.

Dish the sour cream into a bowl. (Fat-free sour cream can be used.) Add some of the hot broth from the pan. Stir to mix, then slowly pour this mess back into the pan.

When the cream has been incorporated into the sauce, dump the cooked noodles into a large lipped dish, top with the chicken and pour the sauce over all.

Ground Turkey Spaghetti Sauce

- 1 pound ground turkey
- 4 cloves garlic, minced
- 2 tablespoons olive oil
- 2 large carrots, chopped
- 1 large onion, chopped
- 1 can (46 ounces) V-8 Juice
- 1 can (6 ounces) tomato paste
- 1 can (28 ounces) chopped canned tomatoes
- 3 tablespoons ketchup
- 1½ teaspoons oregano, crumbled
- 1½ teaspoons basil, crumbled
- 2 teaspoons chili powder

Saute turkey until it begins to brown. Add garlic, onions and carrots and cook 4 minutes. Combine with all other ingredients and simmer for 2 hours.

Makes 6 cups.

You can freeze leftover sauce.

Calcutta Chicken

- 1 cup plain yogurt
- ¼ cup lime juice
- 2 tablespoons canola oil
- 3 garlic cloves garlic, minced
- 1 tablespoon minced ginger root
- 1 teaspoon curry powder
- 1 teaspoon salt
- ½ teaspoon ground cumin
- ½ teaspoon dry mustard
- ½ teaspoon cayenne pepper
- ½ teaspoon black pepper
- ¼ teaspoon turmeric
- 8 chicken thighs

Moosh together all the ingredients except the clucker. Skin the thighs and toss them into a large dish. Add the yogurt mixture and moosh everything around again. Cover and refrigerate the chicken overnight.

An hour before you decide to get hungry, preheat the oven to 350 degrees.

Spread a layer of aluminum foil over the bottom of a large oven dish. Top with the yogurt-coated chicken pieces. Cover the dish with a second sheet of foil and shove into the oven for 40 minutes.

Remove top foil, pour off any excess liquid, then return the uncovered dish to the oven for 15 minutes. Finally, turn the oven heat to broil and briefly brown the thighs on both sides.

You can serve this with rice, but as long as the oven is going to be turned on for an hour, I usually accompany the chicken with oven-browned potatoes.

Quarter the spuds and coat in olive oil. Sprinkle an oven dish with salt, top with the potatoes, sprinkle the tops with salt and pepper and bake for an hour, turning once.

Sage-Garlic Chicken

- 8 fat or 12 medium chicken thighs
- 6 sage leaves (or 1 teaspoon powdered)
- 1 bay leaf
- 8 cloves garlic, peeled but whole
- 1 teaspoon rosemary
- Lots of ground pepper
- Hot pepper flakes to taste
- ¾ cup white wine
- ¼ cup chicken stock
- Salt

If you want, you can remove the skin from the chicken before soaking in cold salted water for half an hour or so. Drain and plunk the thighs into a large skillet with the other ingredients. Simmer covered for 45 minutes. With a spatula, wooden spoon or other blunt instrument squish the garlic into the pan sauces.

Serves 4 with buttered noodles or grits.

A Boiled Bird Feast

- 1 turkey breast
- 4 cups chicken broth
- 4 cups water
- 2 carrots, cut in hunks
- 1 large onion, peeled and sliced thick
- Handful of celery tops
- 1 clove garlic, peeled and halved

Yup, you can produce a low-fat Thanksgiving dinner if you remove the skin from the turkey breast before cooking it like this:

After removing the skin from the breast, fit everything into a large pot.

The liquid should cover the breast. If it doesn't, quite, then turn the turkey breast side down. The other end of the bird doesn't need much cooking.

Bring the pan liquid to a boil, reduce heat and simmer the bird, covered, for 45 minutes. Turn off the heat and, still covered, let the turkey sit in that bath for another hour. It will still be hot when you slice it. It will also be tender, moist and flavorful, although it may look like one of the Seahawks' secondhand footballs.

Strain and freeze the cooking broth. Then when you are down to your last fistful of turkey meat, thaw the stock and bring to a boil with diced carrots and dried noodles for, oh, about 10 minutes or so. Add some frozen peas and the turkey meat, and when the soup is simmering again it's ready to eat.

Oh, yeah, the turkey dinner. To the oven-cooked slices of meat serve unstuffed stuffing.

Sloppy Toms

- 1¼ pounds ground turkey breast
- 1 onion, chopped
- 1 green pepper, chopped
- 1 cup barbecue sauce
- 1 teaspoon liquid smoke
- 1 minced clove garlic
- ½ teaspoon Cajun spice mixture
- ½ teaspoon lemon pepper
- 1 cup water

For this recipe, and for patties, use coarse-grind, low-fat breast meat instead of some in-house ground-turkey special. I usually buy the Turkey Store brand.

Moosh together in a large skillet the turkey, onion and green pepper. Cook until the onions are soft then add all the other ingredients. (I always have a can of Tony Chachere's Creole Seasoning on hand, but if you don't, you can substitute seasoned salt.)

Simmer this mixture 30 minutes or until most of the liquid has boiled away and you have a thick meat mixture. Serve in toasted hamburger buns; should make six sandwiches.

Unstuffed Stuffing

- ¼ cup canola oil
- 1 cup minced onion
- ½ pound mushrooms, halved and sliced thin
- 2 tablespoons port wine
- 12 sage leaves (or 1 teaspoon dried)
- 1 teaspoon dried basil
- ½ cup minced celery
- 1 loaf Italian bread
- 2 eggs, lightly beaten
- 1½ cups chicken broth
- ¼ cup minced parsley

You can use butter in place of canola oil. Or you can use the oil and add Butter Buds to the finished product.

I used a round loaf of Italian bread. You don't want the heavy loaf with the thick crust. Because what you do is to break up the bread with your hands, scatter across a baking pan and toast in a 350-degree oven for 15 minutes, stirring twice.

OK, butter an 8-by-4-inch loaf pan. Butter one side of a 15-inch sheet of waxed paper. Fit the ungreased side into the loaf pan and let the rest of the paper drape over the sides.

Heat the oil in a skillet and saute the onions three minutes. Add the mushrooms and cook until the moisture they exude has cooked away. Slurp in the wine, add the herbs and stir-cook another 2 minutes.

Dump this mess into a large bowl with the bread, celery, eggs, chicken broth and the parsley. Add salt and pepper to taste.

Mix thoroughly, let sit five minutes, then mix again.

Pack the stuffing into the loaf pan. Fold the excess waxed paper over the top and push down lightly to achieve a firm loaf.

Pour two cups of hot water into a baking pan or dish. Put the loaf pan into the water and shove the baking pan into a preheated 250-degree oven. Cook one hour.

Remove the top layer of waxed paper and invert the loaf on a platter. Peel away the remaining waxed paper and boy, are you going to like this stuffing, which will serve four to six, preferably with gravy and the sliced turkey.

This is a great Thanksgiving meal but if Squanto and friends show up at the last minute, they'd better be bringing a tuna casserole with them.

China Burgers

- 1¼ pounds ground turkey meat
- 1 tablespoon peeled ginger root
- 1¼ tablespoons Chinese barbecue sauce
- 1 tablespoon soy sauce
- 1 tablespoon sherry
- 2 green onions, chopped

Cut the ginger root into tiny bits and mix with all the other ingredients.

Use low-fat, coarse ground turkey breast meat. Form five patties and either fry or broil, serving inside hamburger buns with extra Chinese barbecue sauce on the side.

Smoked Chicken

Wash a whole chicken or chicken breasts and rub with salt. Steam or microwave until done. Let cool.

Ignite coals in a covered barbecue. Firmly pack three-quarters of a cup of brown sugar in a measuring cup, then scatter this sugar over an aluminum pan, or a double-thick layer of foil, turned up at the edges. Put the pan on the coals, put the whole chicken or pieces on the BBQ rack and close the lids and all vents. In 20 minutes the chicken should have a nice color and flavor.

Mole Chicken

- 16 chicken thighs
- 2 tablespoons cooking oil
- 4 cloves garlic, minced
- 3 fresh tomatoes, chopped
- 3 jalapenos, diced
- 2 peeled onions, chopped
- ½ cup raisins
- ¼ cup almonds
- 2 wheat tortillas, broken up
- 2 tablespoons chili powder
- 2 tablespoons sesame seeds
- 1 teaspoon salt
- 1 teaspoon cinnamon
- ½ teaspoon ground cloves
- 1 cup fresh cilantro leaves
- ¼ teaspoon pepper
- 1 ounce unsweetened chocolate
- 3½ cups chicken broth

Into a food processor or blender dump the garlic, tomatoes, jalapenos, onions, raisins, almonds, tortillas, chili powder, sesame seeds, salt, cinnamon, cloves, pepper and cilantro. Process until all ingredients have been incorporated into a sauce. Pour this mess into a large pot, add three cups chicken broth and chocolate. Heat until chocolate melts, then remove pot from the heat.

In the hot oil brown eight chicken thighs at a time (skinned or unskinned, as you wish) on both sides, then dump into a large pot.

When all the chicken is cooked and in the pot add the last half-cup of chicken broth and saute gently, covered, about 20 minutes.

Remove chicken and juices to a casserole. Pour the mole sauce over the top and shove into a 325-degree oven for a final 30 minutes. This should serve five to eight guests, depending upon the size of the thighs. It should be accompanied by cooked rice or noodles.

Father's Day Feast

- 2 Cornish game hens
- 1 tablespoon minced ginger root
- 3 cloves garlic, minced
  Cayenne pepper to taste
  Salt, pepper
- ¼ cup soy sauce
- 2 tablespoons sherry
- 2 teaspoons vinegar
- 2 tablespoons molasses
- ¼ cup honey
- ⅓ cup chopped onion
- 1 4-ounce can mushroom stems and pieces
  Bread crumbs
  Chicken broth
  Olive oil

Thaw the hens, remove the little paper sack inside that holds the bird's innards in a neat little bundle. (Is Mother Nature amazing, or what!?)

Mix the ginger, garlic, cayenne and salt and pepper. Carefully shove some of this mixture underneath the breast skin of both birds. Heat a tablespoon of oil in a pan and add the remaining ginger-garlic mixture. Cook for about 30 seconds. Add the combined soy sauce, sherry, vinegar, molasses and honey.

Bring to a boil and remove from heat.

In a skillet saute the onions in a bit of oil, until soft. Coarsely chop the mushrooms and do the same to the raw livers from the sack. Add to the pan with the onions and cook until the liver is no longer pink. Remove from heat and mix in some dry bread crumbs. Add a few dribbles of chicken broth to moisten this mess, which you are supposed to stuff inside each washed-and-dried bird.

If you don't like livers, feed 'em to the cat and simply add more crumbs and more broth to the dressing. You could also add some slivered almonds, if you wish.

When the birds are stuffed, tie the drumsticks together with a bit of string.

OK, plunk the birds in an oven dish and paint with olive oil. Shove into a preheated 350-degree oven. After 30 minutes remove the birds and paint with the soy-sherry mixture, then return to the oven. Repeat this process every 10 minutes or so (if you run out of liquid there will be plenty in the bottom of the oven dish).

After an hour and 15 minutes of total cooking time, remove birds and let stand for 5 minutes. Remove string and serve, maybe with some minted peas. If you like, you can peel and quarter some potatoes, coat them with olive oil, sprinkle with salt and plunk in another pan next to the birds for the full cooking time.

The man in your family can probably eat a whole, stuffed bird by himself.

The kids will probably settle for half a hen. You might want to double this recipe for a large family.

Turkey Meat Loaf

    2 tablespoons canola oil
    1 onion, minced
    1 carrot, shredded
    ¼ cup green onions, minced with green tops
    ½ cup chopped celery
    2 cloves garlic, minced
    1 teaspoon ginger root, minced (or
    ½ teaspoon dried ginger)
    1 cup chili sauce
    1 tablespoon brown sugar
    ¼ cup soy sauce
    1 tablespoon chili powder
    2 large eggs
    2 pounds ground turkey
    1 cup Italian-style seasoned bread crumbs

Heat the oil in a skillet, dump in the onion, carrot, green onions, celery, garlic and ginger. Cook, stirring, for about 5 minutes.

Dump the ground turkey into a large bowl. (Use a top brand of low-fat ground turkey. This will still be a cheap meal.) Crack the eggs on top of the meat (you can use egg substitute), then add the chili sauce, sugar, soy, chili powder and the veggies.

Moosh everything around with your hands. Add the bread crumbs and moosh again until thoroughly combined.

In a large oven dish, form a loaf about 6 by 12 inches. Shove into a 375-degree oven for an hour. Remove dish from oven and let stand 10 minutes before you slice the loaf.

One Dish Dinner for Dummies

    8 chicken breast halves
    5 large carrots
    5 medium potatoes
    1 medium onion
    1 16-ounce bottle zesty Italian dressing
    1 pound broccoli
    1 green pepper
    ½ pound fresh mushrooms

Scrape the carrots and cut into chunks. Wash the potatoes and cut into inch-sized hunks, peeled or unpeeled, to your preference. Thinly slice the onion and cut the seeded green pepper into squares. Thickly slice the mushrooms. Remove the florets from the broccoli and reserve. Peel and thinly slice the stalks.

OK, lay the uncooked breasts out in a large buttered casserole. Sprinkle with salt and pepper. Dump the carrots on top, then the sliced onion, then the sliced broccoli stalks, then the potatoes. Pour the dressing over the top, seal the casserole with foil and shove into a 375-degree oven for one hour.

Remove casserole, turn the breasts, and toss in the green pepper, the broccoli florets and the mushrooms. Cover again and return to oven for 30 minutes or until the potatoes and carrots are done. This should serve six to eight guests.

Golf Balls

    1¼ pounds ground turkey breast
    ½ cup onion, minced
    1 large clove garlic, put through a press
    1 teaspoon salt
    1 teaspoon chili powder
    1 teaspoon ground sage
    Pinch of cayenne pepper

Combine all the ingredients, mix well with your hands, then form into 1-inch-round balls. Lightly spray an oven pan and lay out the turkey balls.

Shove into a 400-degree oven. Check after 20 minutes to see if they are cooked. Avoid overcooking. Serve with Duffer's Gravy.

Duffer's Gravy

    4 tablespoons canola oil or butter
    4 tablespoons flour
    2 cups beef broth
    ½ pound fresh mushrooms
    ½ cup minced green onions
    ½ cup red wine
    1 teaspoon Kitchen Bouquet
    Black pepper

Heat the oil or butter in a saucepan, then slowly stir in the flour. When smooth, stir-cook this mixture 2 minutes, then slowly stir in the beef broth.

While the broth is thickening (stirring occasionally), chop up 3 or 4 mushrooms into small bits. Thickly slice the rest of them.

When the sauce has thickened, add the mushrooms, onions and wine. Simmer 5 minutes, then add the Kitchen Bouquet, the black pepper and the meatballs.

Simmer another 5 minutes and this should serve four golfers with handicaps ranging between 16 and 66.

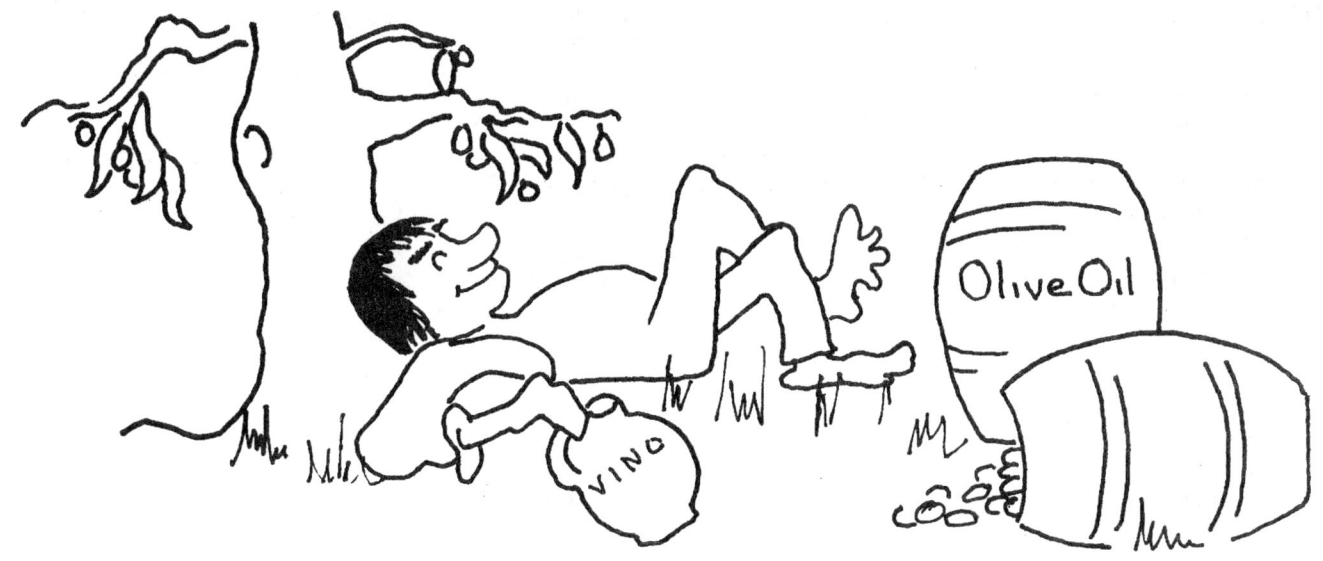

BEEF AND PORK

Possibly somebody from Italy – the land of impassioned eloquence and large families – could explain a term like "almost pregnant." After all, the Italians sold the world a concept of virginity on two levels.

There is a plain and simple virgin. Even more esteemed, however, is the "extra virgin."

Of course we are talking about olive oil, the foundation of the Italian diet. Olive oil recently has been rediscovered by nutritional scientists and is at least partially credited for the good health and longevity of people living in Mediterranean lands.

But there is olive oil. And then there is olive oil.

The "extra virgin" variety is pressed from olives hand-picked from the trees, stone crushed and cold pressed to produce a product with acidity of under 1 percent.

"Virgin" oil is usually produced from older olives, collected after they have fallen from the tree, with somewhat higher acidity.

The term "pure olive oil" is as confusing and misleading as the concepts of extra-virginity and partial pregnancy. Oil earning this label has been deacidified, decolorized and deodorized by chemical means. Next week we may also learn that "pure olive oil" is actually produced from prune pits.

I'm also confused by the instructions Italian chefs impart regarding the proper use of olive oils. Some claim the unique flavor of an extra-virgin product from Umbria or Veneto can only be fully appreciated when savored cold, on a salad or atop sliced tomatoes. And they suggest you save it for such use.

Others instruct their students to use the superior and expensive product to saute seafood, to toss with cooked pasta or to lubricate farm tractors.

I might also use it to brown a pork loin, to saute some pork chops or in cooking up a batch of onions, to serve with some grilled liver.

Meat doesn't have to be eliminated from your diet. But if you have a choice pick a lean flank steak over a well-marbeled T-bone, a lean pork roast as a substitute for spare ribs, or a stir-fry dish which doesn't require much meat.

Roasted Pork Loin

- 2 tablespoons olive oil
- 1 small onion, minced
- 1 clove garlic, minced
- 1 teaspoon dried thyme, crumbled
- 1 teaspoon dried oregano, crumbled
- 1 tablespoon caraway seeds
- 2 teaspoons salt
  Boneless pork loin roast
- 6 small potatoes

This lean cut of meat may range from two to five pounds. Mix together the first seven ingredients, then use your hands to coat the meat on all sides. Let sit in an oven pan refrigerated, all day or overnight, covered.

An hour and a half before dinner, remove pork from the refrigerator and let sit at room temperature while you peel and halve the potatoes and place in a pot. Cover the spuds with water, bring to a boil, then lower heat and simmer 15 minutes. Remove from water and let cool.

Leaving the marinated pork in its oven pan, rub the potatoes with olive oil, salt and pepper and then lay them around the roast. Shove the pan into a preheated 350-degree oven for about an hour, or until a meat thermometer reaches 185 degrees. Tent the meat with foil and let sit 10 minutes on a carving board, returning the pan and potatoes to the oven. Carve the meat and serve with the spuds.

If you want some low-fat gravy, heat a cup of beef broth in a saucepan while the meat is coasting. Measure two tablespoons of Wondra Flour into a quarter cup of water. When smooth, stir this muck into the broth and simmer until it thickens. Add a few drops of Kitchen Bouquet to color and flavor the gravy.

This meal should serve four to six, depending upon the size of the roast.

Glacier Bay Beef

- 1½ pound thin cut eye of round steak
- 1 egg
- 3 tablespoons milk
  Seasoned Italian bread crumbs
- ½ teaspoon garlic salt
  Olive oil
- ¾ cup beef bouillon
- ½ cup marsala wine
- 2 teaspoons flour

With a genuine Capt. Vancouver autographed belaying pin, whack the round steak between two pieces of waxed paper to flatten. Cut into serving portions.

Mix the egg and milk. Dip the pieces of meat in this mess, then dredge into the bread crumbs (I use Progresso), which have been mixed with the garlic salt.

Over medium heat, saute the meat on both sides in olive oil. While this is happening, mix together the beef broth, marsala and flour.

When the meat is golden brown, remove to a warm oven. Dump the wine mixture into the skillet and boil, stirring, until slightly reduced.

Pour the marsala sauce over the meat and this should serve four, with cooked noodles.

Computer Pork Roast

- 5 pound lean pork roast
- ½ teaspoon fennel seed
- ¼ cup flour
  olive oil
- 2 teaspoons salt
- 1 teaspoon pepper
- ½ teaspoon marjoram
- ½ teaspoon thyme
- ¼ teaspoon nutmeg
- 1 cup dry white wine
- 1 cup chicken broth
- ¾ cup apple juice
- 2 cloves garlic
- 1 cup fat-free sour cream

In a mortar or heavy bowl, crush the fennel seed with the salt. Add the flour, pepper and herbs, mix thoroughly and then rub the mixture over all sides of the pork roast.

Coat the bottom of a heavy Dutch oven with a thin layer of olive oil.

Brown the roast on all sides, then glunk into the pot the wine, broth, apple juice and two peeled cloves of garlic.

Put a lid on the pot and shove it into a 325-degree oven 2½ or 3 hours.

Remove the pork to a warm dish, and over a burner boil the pot liquid until it is reduced by half. Remove from heat, skim off the fat and stir in the sour cream.

Slice the pork, pass the gravy, and I like this served with browned potatoes, which you should rub with butter, sprinkle with salt and pepper and then shove uncovered into the oven for the last 75 minutes the pork roast is cooking.

Panhandle Pork Chops

- 4 chops
  Flour and olive oil
- 1 tablespoon paprika
- 1 small onion, chopped
- 1 clove garlic, minced
- ½ teaspoon thyme
- 1 cup white wine
- 2 tablespoons Dijon mustard
  Salt, pepper

I use Dijon mustard in this recipe because I am partial to old French westerns, particularly those that co-starred Brigitte Bardot.

Dredge the chops in flour and brown on both sides in oil. Add the onion, garlic, thyme, paprika and wine and simmer the chops covered until done. That should take about 30 minutes but check once or twice. You don't want to overcook the pork.

Remove the chops to a platter. Stir the mustard into the pan juices and add salt and pepper to taste. Spoon this mess over the chops.

Georgian Stew

- 3 tablespoons olive oil
- 2 onions, chopped
- 1½ pound lean beef chunks
- ½ cup flour
- 2 teaspoons freshly ground black pepper
- salt
- dry white wine
- 4 tomatoes, peeled and chopped
- 2 tablespoons tomato paste
- 1 teaspoon coriander
- 2 teaspoons paprika
- 1/8 teaspoon cayenne pepper
- ¼ cup fresh cilantro, chopped
- ¼ cup fresh parsley, chopped
- ¼ cup fresh basil, chopped

If you don't have fresh basil then use canned Italian chopped tomatoes with basil.

In a heavy kettle heat the oil and saute the onions until soft. Remove. Dump the flour, pepper and salt into a paper sack and shake with the beef cubes to coat them. Add the beef to the pot and brown.

Return the onions to the pot and cover ingredients with white wine (something inexpensive like Gallo chardonnay by the jug.) Cover the pot and shove into a 300-degree oven for an hour. Or you can simmer the stew on top of the stove for the same amount of time.

Remove lid from pot and add the tomatoes, tomato paste, the coriander, paprika and cayenne. Simmer until meat is tender, possibly another 45 minutes, adding more wine or water if needed. Add the parsley, cilanto and basil and simmer another 10 minutes.

Add salt if needed and this should serve four or more, over freshly cooked noodles.

To reduce fat, refrigerate the stew after cooking, then skim off any fat before reheating.

Last Best Steak

- 1 large flank steak
- 1 cup chili sauce
- ¼ cup soy sauce
- 2 tablespoons Worcestershire sauce
- 2 tablespoons molasses
- ½ teaspoon chili powder
- 1 tablespoon minced onion
- ½ teaspoon liquid smoke
- ¼ teaspoon garlic powder
- Salt, pepper

In a pan mix the last nine ingredients. Simmer this muck about 5 minutes, then pour over a flank steak and let it marinate the meat for about 2 hours, turning once or twice. Broil or barbecue and thin slice on the diagonal.

Pecos Parmesan Steak

- 2½ pounds thick-cut round steak
- 2 tablespoons flour
- 1 teaspoon season salt
- ½ teaspoon paprika
- ½ teaspoon instant coffee powder
- ¼ teaspoon garlic powder
- 2 tablespoons olive oil
- ½ cup minced onion
- ½ cup beef bouillon
- ½ cup dry white wine
- ½ cup freshly grated Parmesan
- 2 tablespoons low-fat mayonnaise

With a sharp knife or a dentist's probe, score the steak deeply on both sides.

Mix together the flour, season salt, paprika, coffee powder and garlic powder. Rub well into both sides of the meat.

Heat the oil in a heavy skillet. Brown meat well on both sides. Add the onion, bouillon and wine. Cover the pan tightly and simmer until the meat is tender, about 1 ½ hours. (Check occasionally to be sure the liquids haven't cooked away.)

Remove meat from pan juices and if the gravy needs thickening stir in 1 teaspoon cornstarch mixed into 1 tablespoon water.

Mix the grated Parmesan with the mayo. Spread over the meat and shove the round steak under a broiler just until glazed and brown. Top with the pan gravy.

This should serve 6 cowpokes with lots of mashed spuds on the side.

Frankly Flank

- 1 large flank steak
- Soy sauce
- 1 teaspoon thyme
- ¼ cup chopped green onions
- ¼ cup red wine
- ½ cube of butter (or
- ¼ cup olive oil and Butter Buds)
- Salt and pepper

Paint the steak on both sides with soy sauce. Sprinkle well with salt and pepper. Add the thyme, crumbled, and let the steak stand an hour. (Unless it wants to lie down.) Brush the meat a second time with soy, then shove under an oven broiler until rare (about 4 minutes per side.)

While this is happening, combine in a saucepan the wine and green onions. Bring to a boil, then toss in the butter and add salt to taste.

Carve the steak in thin diagonal slices and serve with the wine sauce, maybe with some twice-baked potatoes.

(For twice-baked potatoes: Bake them an hour in a 400-degree oven. Slice open the top of each spud, spoon the insides of the potato into a bowl and add salt, cheddar cheese, sour cream and chopped green onions. Moosh everything around with a fork, spoon back into the potato shells and return to the oven until hot.)

Onion-Flavored Flank

- ½ cup chopped onion
- 1 tablespoon olive oil
- 1 teaspoon sesame oil
- 2 tablespoons soy sauce
- 2 tablespoons honey
- 2 tablespoons orange juice
- 1 large clove garlic, minced
- dried red pepper flakes, to taste
- 1 flank steak (1 ½ to 2 pounds)

Dump the first eight ingredients into a bowl. Lay the steak out in a flat dish and cut thin diagonal slices in it with a sharp knife. Pour the marinade over the top. Let the meat sit refrigerated in this mess all day or overnight, turning twice.

An hour before you plan to cook, remove the meat from the cooler, allowing it to come to room temperature. Scrape off the onion, then barbecue or broil the steak on both sides, basting twice with the marinade, for about eight minutes total, or until medium rare. Carve thin slices on the diagonal and this should serve four, with a tossed salad and baked potatoes.

Navajo Stew

- 2 pounds lean beef chunks
- 2 tablespoons olive oil
- 2 onions, sliced
- 4 cloves garlic, minced
- 1 cup chopped celery
- 2½ cups tomatoes
- 1 teaspoon salt
- Freshly ground pepper
- ½ teaspoon thyme
- 1 cup frozen peas
- 12 small carrots
- 1 can (1 pound) tiny onions
- 6 potatoes, peeled and quartered
- 1 cup red wine
- ½ cup flour
- ½ teaspoon Kitchen Bouquet

Brown the beef chunks in the hot oil. Then add the sliced onions, garlic, celery, tomatoes (which have first been put through a blender), thyme, salt, pepper, wine and 1 ½ cups of water.

Bring to a boil, lower heat, cover and simmer the pot 2 hours.

Add to the pot the potatoes and carrots, and simmer, covered, another 45 minutes.

Drain the baby onions, saving the liquid. Add them and the peas to the pot.

Mix the flour with ¾ cup of the liquid from the canned onions. When smooth, stir into the pot along with the Kitchen Bouquet. Let the stew thicken and this should serve about four.

Scandi Meatballs

- 4 pounds lean ground beef
- 4 eggs or egg substitute
- 1½ cups cracker crumbs
- 1 cup milk
- 1½ teaspoons celery salt
- 1 teaspoon freshly ground pepper
- ¼ teaspoon grated nutmeg
- ½ cup minced onion
- 4 tablespoons butter or olive oil
- ¼ cup flour
- 4 cups beef broth
- Cooked noodles

The secret to great Scandinavian meatballs lies in the grinding. The butcher shop grind isn't good enough. What you have to do is to combine the beef, eggs, cracker crumbs, milk, celery salt, pepper, nutmeg and onion in a heavy-duty mixer or (better yet) in a food processor. Lean on the button until the meat is thoroughly minced and the other ingredients are incorporated.

Wetting your hands repeatedly (gee, isn't this a fun ritual?), you get to pinch off portions of the meat mixture and form into one-inch balls.

Heat the butter or oil and brown the meatballs on all sides, in batches. Remove with a slotted spoon. When the last meatball has been cooked, pour off all but four tablespoons of oil. Mix in the flour, then slowly add the beef broth. Bring to a boil and simmer until the gravy thickens. Then return the meatballs to the pan or pot, reduce heat and simmer everything, covered, for 15 minutes.

This should serve eight generously, over noodles.

Pork Vindaloo

- 1½ pounds lean pork
- 4 cloves garlic
- ¾ cup white wine vinegar
- 2 tablespoons coriander seeds
- 1 tablespoon chili powder
- ¼ teaspoon cayenne
- 8 peppercorns
- 1 tablespoon cumin seeds
- 1 tablespoon mustard seeds
- ½ teaspoon powdered ginger

In a blender puree the last nine ingredients. Use this as a bath for the pork, cut into 1-inch hunks.

When ready to cook, dump the pork and marinade into a saucepan along with ¼ cup water. Cover and simmer slowly for 90 minutes. Remove cover and simmer a final 15 minutes (unless the sauce has already been cooked down sufficiently.) Serves four with steamed rice.

Capt. Rafferty's Loaf

- 1½ pounds leanest ground beef
- 1 medium onion, peeled and chopped
- 2 cloves garlic, minced
- 1¼ cups Italian bread crumbs
- 2 eggs (or equivalent egg substitute)
- ⅓ cup tomato juice
- 2 teaspoons lemon juice
- ½ teaspoon dried basil
- ½ teaspoon dried oregano
- 1¼ teaspoons salt
- ¼ teaspoon allspice
- ¼ teaspoon cayenne pepper (or to taste)
- ½ cup catsup
- Tabasco to taste

Saute the onions and garlic in a bit of oil, just until they have softened. Dump into a bowl along with the beef, crumbs, eggs, tomato juice, lemon juice, basil, oregano, salt, allspice and cayenne. With clean hands execute a stranglehold on this ominous lump and keep squeezing and kneading until meatloaf ingredients are well mixed.

Stuff ingredients into an oiled loaf pan (it should fill to within ¾ inch of the top). Shove into a 350 oven for an hour.

Mix the catsup with tabasco to your preferred to degree of heat. Remove loaf from oven, top with this mixture, then return to oven for 20 minutes. Remove loaf again and let it coast for at least five minutes before carving.

Ancient Healing Stir Fry

- ⅓ cup soy sauce
- 2 tablespoons sherry
- 3 cloves garlic, minced
- 1 teaspoon red pepper flakes
- 4 tablespoons cornstarch
- 1 pound beef flank or sirloin
- 4 tablespoons canola oil
- 4 cups assorted vegetables
- ½ cup beef broth
- ⅓ cup Chinese barbecue sauce
- ¼ cup black bean sauce
- 2 tablespoons wine
- cornstarch

Usually a stir-fry is designed to clean out the vegetable bin in your refrigerator, so use whatever is on hand to make up the four cups. A typical assortment would be a cup and a half of broccoli florets, a cup of cauliflower buds, a half-cup of sliced carrots, a half-cup of green pepper in 1-inch squares and a half-cup of sliced water chestnuts.

First combine the soy sauce, sherry, garlic and a half teaspoon of red pepper flakes and moosh this around with the meat, which has been thinly sliced. Let this mess sit in the refrigerator for an hour or so.

When ready to cook, heat two tablespoons of oil in a large skillet. If you are using the veggies suggested above, add the broccoli, cauliflower and carrots at this point and stir-fry 3 or 4 minutes. Remove to a warm dish.

Add a tablespoon of oil to the skillet and saute the green pepper for a minute. Add the water chestnuts, cook another minute and toss them on the plate, too.

Add another tablespoon or so of the canola oil to the pan and stir-fry drained meat strips. Dump the veggies into the pan with the meat.

Mix together the beef broth, Chinese barbecue sauce (you can find it in oriental grocery stores), bean sauce, wine, another half teaspoon of red pepper flakes and two tablespoons cornstarch. Add to the pan and stir-fry until thickened. Cover, cook 2 minutes more, then serve up on a platter. With rice this should serve four.

Shiver My Liver

- 1 tablespoon flour
- ½ teaspoon chili powder
- Salt
- Pepper
- 6 thin slices calf liver
- 1 tablespoon oil
- 4 tablespoons red wine
- 1 tablespoon minced green onion
- 2 cloves garlic, chopped
- Pinch each of thyme, basil and sage
- ¼ cup beef broth

Mix the salt, pepper and flour with the chili powder and use to coat the liver lightly. Saute on both sides in the hot oil, 1 to 2 minutes total.

Remove the liver slices to a warm dish.

To the skillet add the wine, green onions and garlic. Cook a minute or two, then add the herbs and beef broth. When it reaches a simmer, pour it over the liver slices and this will serve three liver lovers or 132 people who aren't.

Liver Trattoria

- 1 pound thin-sliced beef or calve's liver
- olive oil
- marsala wine
- 1 clove garlic, minced
- ½ teaspoon Italian herbs
- Freshly ground pepper
- ⅓ cup chopped green onions

Lay liver in a rimmed dish and pour marsala over it to cover. Stir in the garlic, herbs and lots of freshly ground pepper. Let sit for an hour.

At dinner time, remove liver from marinade and dry with paper towels. Saute the liver in a skillet with hot olive oil for about 2 minutes per side. Remove to a warm dish. Slop the leftover marinade into the skillet, add the green onion, boil until reduced by half and pour over the liver.

Java Ginger Beef

- 1 pound beef flank steak
- 1 tablespoon cornstarch
- 1 tablespoon soy sauce
- 1 tablespoon sesame oil
- 1 tablespoon Dijon mustard
- ½ teaspoon red pepper flakes
- 1 heaping tablespoon peeled and shredded fresh ginger root
- 1 teaspoon salt
- 2 tablespoons cooking oil
- 2 teaspoons sugar
- ¼ cup sherry
- 2 cups chopped cilantro

Slice the flank against the grain, as thin as possible. It's easier to do this if the meat is almost frozen.

In a small bowl, mix the cornstarch, soy, sesame oil, mustard and red pepper flakes. Dump this onto the meat slices, mix thoroughly with a chopstick until all the meat is coated with the sauce, then let sit refrigerated for an hour or so.

Mix the ginger with the salt. After a half hour, squeeze as much moisture as you can out of the ginger. Dissolve the sugar in the sherry.

OK, heat the oil in a large skillet. When hot, stir-fry the marinated meat until no longer pink. Add the ginger and stir-fry 30 seconds more. Stir in the cilantro and the sherry mixture, gloop it all around, and serve with some cooked noodles or rice.

This should be enough beef for four served with side dishes.

California Liver

- 4 avocados
- 1/3 cup plus 1 tablespoon lemon juice
- 2 tablespoons olive oil
- 4 tablespoons butter
- 12 slices calf liver
- ½ cup flour
- 1 teaspoon salt
- ½ teaspoon pepper
- ½ cup beef broth
- ½ teaspoon thyme

The avocado should not be rock hard or too soft. Peel, seed and slice the little buggers, then sprinkle with one tablespoon of lemon juice. The liver slices (to serve six) should be thin cut and will weigh about a pound and a half total.

Mix some salt and pepper into the flour and dredge both the liver and avocado slices. Coat the bottom of a large skillet with olive oil. Saute the liver and avocado very quickly over a medium-hot fire, in two batches if needed, and remove when cooked to dish in a warm oven. The way to screw up this dish is by overcooking.

In the same skillet, melt the butter. When it sizzles, stir in 1/3 cup lemon juice, the broth and thyme. Bring to a boil then pour over the liver and avocado and serve with toast slices.

Sweetbreads for Sweethearts

- 1 pound veal sweetbreads
- 1 tablespoon vinegar
- 1 teaspoon salt
- 1 tablespoon lemon juice
- 3 tablespoons butter or oil
- ¼ cup minced ham
- ¼ cup minced celery
- ¼ cup minced onion
- ¼ cup minced carrot
- ½ pound mushrooms, chopped
- ¼ teaspoon thyme
- Salt, pepper to taste
- ¾ cup dry white wine
- 1 cup beef broth
- 1 tablespoon ketchup

Some supermarket clerks may give you an odd look if you ask for a pound of sweetbreads. But the better butchers carry them, fresh or frozen. For this recipe I got mine from Don and Joe, who are not members of the Moran Mob in Chicago. They run a first-rate Pike Place meat market.

Fresh or thawed, wash the sweetbreads in cold water, then soak an hour in water mixed with the vinegar.

Drain the sweetbreads and dump into a saucepan with more cold water, salt and the lemon juice. Bring to a boil and simmer five minutes. Cool under running water.

Break the sweetbreads up with your hands into bite-sized or slightly larger pieces, discarding any tough membrane. (This is not the romantic part of the meal. That starts later.)

In a skillet saute the sweetbreads in butter just until brown on both sides. Remove to an open casserole, one just big enough to accommodate the nuggets in one layer.

To the skillet add the celery, carrot, onion, ham and mushrooms and cook for about 4 minutes, adding more butter or oil as needed. Stir in the thyme plus salt and pepper to taste. Scatter this mess over the sweetbreads.

To the same skillet add the wine and beef broth. Boil until reduced by half. Stir in the ketchup. Pour this mess over the sweetbreads and veggies.

Shove the uncovered casserole into a 325-degree oven for 40 minutes.

Now comes the sexy part. Serves two over crisp toast, with a salad on the side.

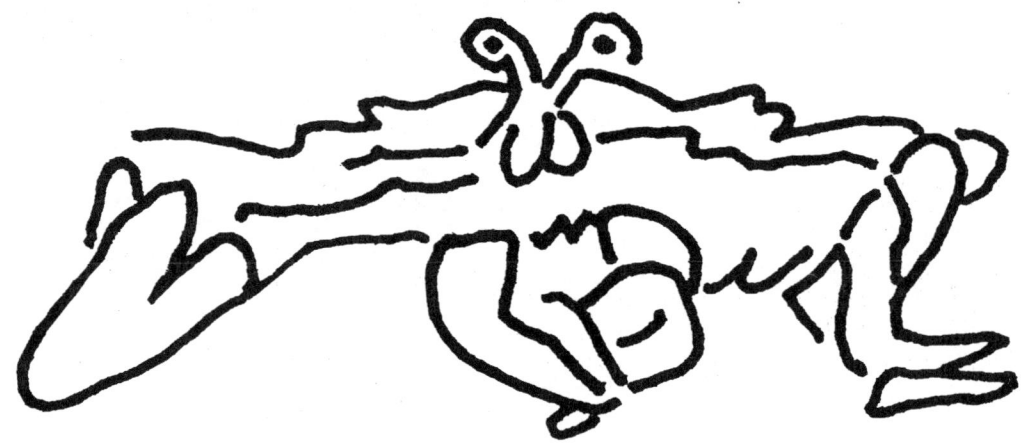

SEAFOOD

It's unlikely you'll see this dialogue repeated in your favorite Harlequin novel. But it's a greeting a lot of American men receive after a day out in the business and industrial jungle. Our hero staggers into his lover's waiting arms, plants a passionate kiss upon her lips and hears her gasp, "You had garlic for lunch. And onions, too, unless I miss my guess."

That's negative reinforcement and plays havoc with the libido. It's time those words of greeting were revised.

What Your Significant Other should say, after that passionate smooch, is this: "Gee you smell healthy today." And it's true. You do.

According to the latest medical evidence, garlic raises the levels of "good" cholesterol in the blood and lowers the level of "bad." And onion seems to have the same effect. As a consequence, a lot of health experts are recommending consumption of one clove of garlic, or half an onion, each day.

I suppose you could take a garlic pill, but give me a break! That makes about as much sense as asking your loved one to hand you a kiss capsule and a glass of water when you get home from work.

The beneficial effects of garlic and onion are enhanced by their flavors and aromas, which sharpen the appetite, encouraging you to consume other healthy items like penne with red pepper and anchovies or a spicy fillet of sauteed snapper.

Yeah, spices are also important to your good health. They soothe, rather than irritate, the angry stomach and put zing into your kisses, especially in sexy seafood dishes. Or haven't you heard how many eggs a salmon lays after even the most casual relationship?

Hook, Line, Sinker

- 2 pounds fish fillets
- 1 jar (4 ounces) cocktail onions
- 5 garlic cloves, peeled
- 6 whole peppercorns
- Juice of one lemon
- 1 tablespoon mayonnaise
- Olive oil
- 1 to 2 chipotle chilies
- Salt to taste

Dump the cocktail onions (with the vinegar from the bottle) into a blender along with the garlic, peppercorns, lemon juice and mayonnaise. Blend, then slowly add olive oil with machine running until you have a spreadable sauce. Add one chipotle chili and blend again. Taste to see if the sauce is hot enough. If you have a higher tolerance for fire, add more chili and blend again.

(If you can't find or don't like chipotle chilies, you could use jalapenos. But it won't be quite the same, Conchita!)

Lay the fillets (cod, snapper or whatever is cheap) out in one layer of an oven dish. Spread the sauce over the top. Shove into a 350-degree oven for 45 minutes to one hour, depending upon the thickness of the fish.

The above formula will cure colds and "flu," enhance your love life and help promote prosperity among the onion, garlic and chili pepper growers of America.

Green Onion Fillets

- 2 pounds fish fillets
- 1 bunch green onions
- 2 green peppers
- 3 tomatoes
- ¼ cup cilantro leaves
- 2 tablespoons olive oil
- 1 lemon sliced
- Garlic salt

Chop the green onions, including the green tops. Char the peppers over a gas or electric burner on the stove, then peel with your hands under cold water and cut the peppers into strips, discarding the seeds. (If you just want to use unpeeled pepper strips and save yourself all that trouble, turn in your written excuse to the office.)

Dunk the tomatoes into boiling water for 10 seconds, then peel and chop.

Lay the fillets out in an oven dish. Sprinkle generously with garlic salt, then top with the onions, green peppers, tomatoes, cilantro, a drizzle of olive oil and the slices of lemon. Bake at 375 degrees for 20 minutes, or until done. Don't overcook. Serves 4.

Far Out Fish

- 1 tablespoon olive oil
- 1 cup fresh wheat bread crumbs
- 1 large clove garlic
- ⅓ cup Dijon mustard
- 4 tablespoons minced fresh basil (or
- 1 teaspoon dried)
- 4 halibut steaks

Heat the oil in a skillet, add the crumbs and garlic and stir-cook until golden. Mix the mustard with the basil. Spread this mess on both sides of the fish, then top with the crumb mixture, pressing to make it stick to the fish.

Bake in a preheated 450-degree oven 10 to 15 minutes or until done. Serve with something we might call:

Love Apple Salsa

- 1½ cups chopped plum tomatoes
- 1 avocado, peeled and chopped
- ¾ cup sweet red pepper, chopped
- ¼ cup minced red onion
- 2 tablespoons fresh cilantro
- 1 tablespoon red wine vinegar
- 1 tablespoon olive oil

Gloop the above ingredients together and serve at room temperature with the fish. If you don't like or can't find fresh cilantro, use parsley instead.

Hornby Island Halibut

- 2 pounds halibut fillets
- Salt, pepper
- 2 tablespoons lemon juice
- ⅓ cup mayonnaise
- 1 teaspoon soy sauce
- ¾ cup Oriental panko or Italian bread crumbs
- ¾ cup slivered almonds

Sprinkle the fillets with salt and pepper. Baste with lemon juice and let stand 15 minutes.

Place fillets in lightly oiled oven dish or pan. Mix soy with mayonnaise and spread over the fish. Coat the fillets with crumbs and lay in pan. Over the top scatter the nuts and press them in so they'll stick to the fish.

Bake in a preheated 350-degree oven from 20 to 30 minutes, depending upon the thickness of the fillets. Serves four to six.

Mint Pesto for Salmon

    2 cups firmly packed mint leaves
    1 tablespoon chopped nuts
    ¼ teaspoon salt
    1 small clove garlic, minced
       Olive oil
    3 tablespoons grated Parmesan cheese

Toss the fresh mint leaves into a food processor or blender along with the salt, garlic and nuts. (I used pine nuts but walnuts are OK.)

Hit the button on your food processor and then slowly add olive oil. Don't process too long or use too much oil. You want a substance that can be spread across the top of a salmon fillet with a knife. Transfer pesto to a dish and stir in the cheese.

Broil salmon or halibut fillets to your liking, then remove to plates, spread with the pesto while the fish is still steaming hot and serve. It's terrific because it cuts the fishy taste, if there was one. This is enough pesto for three portions of fish. Obviously, you can double or triple the recipe if you have enough mint.

Or, you can toss the mint pesto with spaghettini and serve that simply. Or you could add some slices of freshly broiled chicken breast.

Myrtle's Calamari

    1   pound squid
    ¼   pound fettuccine
    ¼   cup olive oil
    3   dried hot red chilies
    ⅓   cup dry white wine
         Handful of chopped parsley
         Freshly grated Parmesan
         Tomato Sauce (recipe follows)

If your squid jig is in the garage for repairs, you can buy the calamari at the Pike Place Market. If you buy it already cleaned, you'll probably only need ¾ of a pound.

Cut the cleaned squid in half-inch rings.

Heat the oil in a skillet along with the dried peppers. After 2 minutes remove and discard the chilies. Toss the squid into the hot oil and stir-cook for about 30 seconds. Add the wine and cook another minute. Add tomato sauce, reduce heat and simmer for 10 minutes. Add the chopped parsley.

Meanwhile, you should have been cooking the pasta in salted boiling water.

Drain it and dump it into the skillet with the sauce.

Toss and serve onto two warm plates, adding freshly grated Parmesan to taste.

The Tomato Sauce:

    8 ounces canned tomato sauce
    1 small fresh tomato, chopped
    2 minced cloves garlic
    ½ teaspoon oregano
    ½ teaspoon basil

Simmer this sauce 10 minutes and add to the squid as described above.

Foiled Trout

The supermarkets usually carry fresh trout about 12 inches in length before you cut off the head and tail. Some people prefer to leave the tail on. You can leave the head on, too, if you don't mind being scrutinized by the fish all the way through supper.

Anyway, plunk each trout on a piece of aluminum foil, pulling the edges up to form a rim. Spread some olive oil or butter inside each fish. Put a large clove of garlic through a press and use the puree to coat the inside of one trout.

Salt the inside of the fish, then slop some white wine in the center and over the top of the fish (2 tablespoons total). Repeat this process for each fish. Then wrap each trout in the foil, leaving a small pocket of air. Crimp the foil so the wine won't leak out.

Plunk the wrapped fish on a rimmed cooking pan and shove into a preheated, 400-degree oven for about 25 minutes. Place an unwrapped trout on each plate. Your guests merely have to peel back the top skin with their dinner knives and dig in. Supply those who want them with hunks of lemon for squeezing. When you have finished half of the fish you can lift the bones out in one piece and discard, then finish your meal.

Seacombe Salmon

    1 cup chicken broth
    ½ teaspoon dried tarragon
    ½ teaspoon thyme leaves
    4 salmon steaks
    1 clove garlic, minced
    1 teaspoon cornstarch
    3 tablespoons minced chives or green onions
       salt, pepper
       lemon wedges

Heat a skillet and add the broth and herbs. Bring to a boil, then remove from stove and distribute salmon steaks over the pan. Reduce heat and simmer the salmon covered 10 to 15 minutes, just until the fish no longer looks raw inside.

Remove steaks to a warm platter and cover with foil.

Dump the garlic into the pan juices and boil until the liquid is reduced by half. Mix the cornstarch with two tablespoons of water and stir into the pan. Stir until the broth thickens and clears. Mix in the chives and pour this sludge over the steaks.

Low Budget Fish Stew

- ¼ cup olive oil
- 1 onion, minced
- ½ teaspoon red pepper flakes
- 1 green bell pepper, chopped
- 3 minced garlic cloves
- 1 tablespoon red wine vinegar
- 1½ cups dry white wine
- 1 can (about 30 oz.) crushed tomatoes
- 1 teaspoon oregano
- 2 tablespoons ketchup
- Sugar to taste
- 2 to 2½ pounds bottomfish fillets

In a soup pot, saute the onion and green pepper in the olive oil, until softened. Add the garlic, vinegar and red pepper flakes. Stir over heat until vinegar cooks away. Add to the pot the wine and oregano. Simmer 5 minutes, then dump in the crushed tomatoes and the ketchup. Taste to see if the sauce needs some sugar. You probably wouldn't want to use more than a teaspoon. Simmer the sauce covered 15 minutes.

Cut the fish fillets (I used previously frozen true cod but snapper is OK) into large hunks and add to the pot. Simmer 5 minutes or just until fish is cooked, then dish up into four large or six small bowls and serve with crusty bread.

Salmon Spuds

- 1 (14 ounce) can red salmon
- 4 baking potatoes
- ½ cup milk
- ¼ cup non-fat sour cream
- ½ cup Parmesan cheese
- ¼ cup minced green onion
- 1 teaspoon dried thyme
- ½ teaspoon salt
- Pepper
- ½ cup frozen peas, thawed

Wash the spuds, rub with oil and prick in several places with a fork. Bake at 400 degrees for an hour.

Cut the tops off the spuds and scoop out the pulp. Mash the potatoes with heated milk. Beat in the Parmesan, onion, thyme, salt and pepper.

Stir in the sour cream, salmon and peas. Stuff the potatoes, mounding the top. Bake stuffed spuds another 15 minutes at 350 degrees.

Sue-Ellen's Salmon Loaf

- 1 one-pound can of salmon, preferably red
- ⅓ cup green pimento olives, sliced
- ¼ cup minced onions
- ½ cup dried Italian bread crumbs
- 2 beaten eggs (or egg substitute)
- ½ teaspoon salt
- ½ teaspoon Tabasco
- ½ teaspoon liquid smoke

All you do is remove and discard skin from canned salmon. Flake it with a fork, then stir in other ingredients. Stuff into small oiled loaf pan. Cook 30 minutes in 350-degree oven. This will give you about 4 servings. Or, double the recipe and oven cook it 35 or 40 minutes in a large loaf pan.

Salmon Cakes

- 3 tablespoons canola oil
- ½ cup chopped onions
- ¼ cup chopped parsley
- 3 cups leftover mashed potatoes
- 1 can (7.5 ounces) red salmon
- Salt to taste
- Cayenne pepper to taste
- 1 egg, beaten
- ½ teaspoon garlic powder
- 1 cup seasoned Italian bread crumbs

You can often buy small cans of red salmon for only about two bucks. Open the can and drain off the liquid.

Saute the onions in the oil, then let cool.

In a bowl, flake the salmon and mix in the mashed potatoes, onions, parsley and garlic powder. Taste to see how much salt and cayenne you want to add. Mix in the egg and bread crumbs.

Mix well and form 3-inch cakes, placing on a large sheet of waxed paper after you have formed each one in your hands. You should have about 10 cakes.

Heat some more canola oil in a large skillet and saute the cakes until browned on both sides. Keep first batch warm in the oven while the rest of the cakes cook.

Aquatic Pork Chops

- 1½ pounds cheap fish fillets
- mayonnaise
- 1 package pork chop coating

This sounds like a mess but it is really pretty good. True cod is a good choice for this dish. Just paint each fillet on both sides with mayo, then coat on both sides with the pork chop coating (there are several different brands on the grocery shelves). Put the fillets in an ungreased pan and cook in preheated 400-degree oven for 10 minutes or until fish flakes with a fork.

Balsamic Salmon

¼ cup balsamic vinegar
2 teaspoons canola oil
½ cup fresh mint leaves, minced
2 tablespoons honey
4 salmon fillet portions
Salt to taste
1 lemon

In an antique apothecary bowl, moosh together the vinegar, honey and oil. Brush the fish with this muck. Shove under a broiler about 8 minutes, basting once with sauce. Salt if you wish.

Remove from broiler and top the fish with minced mint. Serve with lemon wedges.

Limustard Salmon

4 portions of salmon fillet (1 ½ pounds total)
2 tablespoons coarse German mustard
2 limes
Salt, pepper

Peel just the green outside part of the limes and chop. Mix with the mustard and 2 tablespoons juice from the limes. Add salt and pepper to taste.

Coat the fillets with this mess and cook under broiler until done, usually 8 to 10 minutes.

Hawaiian Halibut

Halibut steaks or fillets to serve four
2 limes
1 ripe avocado
1 teaspoon of minced Hawaiian hot pepper (or jalapeno)
1 large green onion, including top, chopped
1 small fresh tomato, chopped
½ cup chopped fresh cilantro leaves

Granted, in Hawaii you are more likely to find swordfish or mahi-mahi in a seafood market counter, and either of those can be substituted.

Mash or chop the peeled avocado and mix with the juice of one lime, plus the pepper, onion and fresh tomato.

Use the other lime for juice to sprinkle over the fish steaks. Broil the halibut or bake at 425 degrees for about 18 minutes. Remove fish to four plates; top with guacamole sprinkled with cilantro.

Snappy Snapper

2 tablespoons canola oil
juice of 1 small lemon
1 tablespoon rosemary
1 pound snapper fillets
1 tablespoon Dijon mustard
⅓ cup tomato sauce
1 tablespoon ketchup
¼ teaspoon Tabasco sauce
2 tablespoons red wine vinegar

In a skillet heat the oil, lemon juice and rosemary until boiling. Add fish fillets and cook 30 seconds on each side. Push fillets to one side of the pan and stir in all the other ingredients, which have first been mixed together in a bowl.

Move fish back to center of pan, reduce heat, cover and poach for about six minutes, or until the fillets flake with a fork.

Along with brown rice and a salad, this will serve four, with the pan sauce spooned over the top of the fish.

Solidarity Squid

1 pound squid rings
¼ cup olive oil
1 onion, thinly sliced
2 green peppers, thinly sliced
1 large clove garlic, minced
1 6-ounce can tomato sauce
⅓ cup red wine
8 large black olives, halved
Salt, pepper

You can usually buy squid cleaned and cut into small rings. If you can't find this product, you may have to clean and skin the squid yourself, in which case you deserve a big tip from the customers.

Heat the oil in a skillet and saute the onion slices until they soften. Add the green pepper strips, garlic and tomato sauce and simmer for about 20 minutes. Add the wine, the olives and the squid and cook another 5 minutes.

Salt and pepper to taste.

This should serve four with rice or noodles.

French Fish

    1   tablespoon brandy
    2   tablespoons lemon juice
    4   tablespoons Dijon mustard
    ½   teaspoon thyme
    ½   teaspoon salt
    4   green onions
    ½   cup chopped parsley
  1½   pounds fish fillets

The last time I prepared this dish I used a couple of inexpensive slabs of true cod, which were on special at my local market.

Combine the brandy, lemon juice, mustard, thyme and salt in a bowl and beat until thoroughly combined. Let this mess sit at least 15 minutes before you proceed with the recipe.

Scatter the chopped green onions (including most of the green tops) over an oven dish. Do the same with the parsley.

Lay out the fish fillets and pour the sauce over all. Lift the fillets to make sure there is sauce underneath.

Then all you have to do is to shove the dish into a preheated 450-degree oven and the fish should be cooked in 15 to 20 minutes, depending upon the thickness of the fillets.

Dijon Sole

    ¾   pound sole fillets
         Dijon mustard
    1   cup grated Parmesan cheese
    ½   cup dry Italian bread crumbs

Lay the fillets out in an oven dish. Spread lightly with mustard, then sprinkle with the crumbs, then top with the Parmesan. Add more crumbs (I use Progresso) and cheese if you think it needs some.

Shove the dish into a preheated 400-degree oven 15-20 minutes, until the cheese is golden and the fish is barely cooked through. Serves two.

Sexual Stereotypes During Snack Time in America

The man in the house might tend to slice some beef from a leftover roast and slap it between two pieces of rye, with mustard and raw onion, for a late-night snack.

His female counterpart gasps in horror, and opts for a few cubes of cheese with a cracker or two.

It would be better for both if they opted for tuna sandwiches. And hold the melted cheddar.

Cheese is one of the most popular high-fat snacks. The average American consumes 26 pounds a year. But the typical block of cheese contains between 65 and 75 per cent fat.

One ounce of extra-sharp cheddar contains approximately 14 grams of fat. That's about twice as much fat as is contained in Jarlsberg, farmer, feta, goat cheese, Havarti light or part-skim mozzarella.

An American cheese sandwich contains about 12 grams of fat, three grams more than are found in a bologna sandwich. A tuna sandwich, by contrast, contains one gram of fat, if you use a non-fat mayonnaise.

Sorry, Charlie.

SHELLFISH

Madison Avenue has a ready explanation for mysterious phenomena that defy laws of physics or chemistry.

"It's gotta be the shoes!"

In this case, I don't think so.

It might be the legs. It could be the dogs. Certainly "vin rouge" has been implicated. But there may not be any single factor explaining why the residents of France survive, prosper and outlive most Americans on a diet that seems to be five parts cheese and two parts whipped cream with pate foie gras filling in the culinary cracks.

It's known as "the French paradox" and the Intermediate Eater recently traveled 3,000 miles through Paris, the Alps, the Riviera, Provence, Burgundy, Normandy and a dozen intermittent stops trying to learn why the French are immune to the laws of nutrition as they are preached in this country.

Along the way we exploded a few myths expounded by nervous celery nibblers in the New World.

"The average Frenchman eats very little meat. It's only the rich who feast like 16th-century counts," American skeptics rationalize.

Wrong. We visited at least 15 large and small-town outdoor markets over a period of 25 days and watched the local shoppers loading up on baseball-sized lumps of goat cheese and generous slabs of liver pate and meat terraine. They were also liable to pick up an armload of sausages before heading to the bakery for an assortment of tarts, cakes and candies.

In the restaurants, everybody seems to be eating four-course meals. Mussels in garlic butter, lamb kidneys in red wine, two kinds of cheese and flan floating in warm chocolate constitutes a typical repast, along with a bottle or two of the local red wine.

I emulated the locals with an enthusiasm bordering on lust, abandoning for the month what is normally a low-fat American diet. Before leaving Seattle I subjected myself to a blood test. The day after I flew back from Paris I took another, out of curiosity and at the suggestion of Alice the Artist. My cholesterol reading was exactly the same as it had been a month before, when I had departed Seattle nibbling on some Ry-Krisp.

How can I explain it?

It wasn't the Hush Puppies I wore. But it might be the poodles. Every Frenchman, and woman, seems to own a poodle. They walk them every day, usually down to the bakery for a few baguettes. Every day, morning and night, the French walk their dogs and their loaves.

Most people residing in villages or cities climb stairs to their apartments. It is not unusual to climb 50 stairs in a city like Nice or Paris. Elevators are nonexistent in 90 percent of the apartments or hotels.

So the French get a lot more exercise than Americans. Their meals are considerable but relaxed, usually spread out over an hour or more. (Even mom and pop grocery stores close from noon to 2 p.m.) The wine is inexpensive, drinkable and is shared by the young and old. I never saw a milk truck in France. I saw a whole lot of wine trucks, making block-by-block deliveries.

Although the French consume a lot of dairy products, they probably eat fewer products containing partially hydrogenated vegetable oils, a curse of the American diet.

Somehow, it all works for the French. And, at least for a month, it worked for me. Surprisingly, I didn't even gain any weight, despite multi-course meals that might have begun with a bowl of Normandy mussels in cream. In this chapter we suggest how such a delicacy can be converted into a low-calorie treat, for the dog-deprived gourmands who don't get nearly enough healthful exercise.

Normandy Mussels for Four

    3   cups dry white wine
    1   rib celery with leaves
    1   clove garlic, chopped
    1   onion, peeled and chopped
    ¾   teaspoon salt
    ¼   teaspoon pepper
    5   pounds mussels, debearded
    1½ cups cream or low-fat evaporated milk
   *5   tablespoons butter
    5   tablespoons flour

Dump the first six ingredients into a large pot, bring to a boil and simmer 15 minutes. While it is simmering, melt the butter in a small saucepan and stir in the flour. When smooth, add the cream in small splashes and stir-cook until it thickens. (Substitute the evaporated milk if you are on a low-fat diet.)

Toss the cleaned mussels into the pot with the wine mixture. Steam covered until the little buggers open. Remove to four large plates. Stir the cream sauce into the pan juices and divide mixture among the four bowls of mussels.

* Some mussel lovers might want to eliminate the butter and flour thickening and add cream or evaporated milk directly to the pan juices before heating and pouring over the mussels.

Herbed Mussels

    4   pounds Penn Cove mussels to serve four
    1   cup dry white wine
    1   cup minced onion
    ½   teaspoon dry thyme
    1   stalk celery, in 2-inch hunks
    ½   cup olive oil
    2   tablespoons red wine vinegar
    1   clove garlic, minced
    ½   teaspoon salt
    1   tablespoon curry powder

Toss the mussels into a large pot. Add the wine, onion, thyme and celery.

In a small saucepan combine the olive oil, vinegar, garlic, salt and curry powder. Put over very low heat but do not allow to boil.

OK, turn up the heat under the mussels. Cook covered, shaking the pot once or twice, until all of the little buggers open up.

Drain the mussels in a colander then dump into a large bowl. Top with the curry sauce, toss the mussels to coat and then let your guests help themselves, along with salad and French bread.

Oven Oysters

    1   jar (10 ounces) oysters
    ¼   cup olive oil (or butter)
    ½   cup Bisquick
    1½ tablespoon yellow corn meal
    ¼   teaspoon paprika
    ¼   teaspoon garlic salt
    ¼   teaspoon black pepper
    2   eggs or egg substitute

Drain the oysters and cut in half if large, then pat 'em dry with paper towels.

Pour the oil into a foil-lined pan. Heat in a 425-degree oven, then remove.

Combine the Bisquick, cornmeal and spices. Lightly beat the eggs.

Dip the oysters in egg, then in crumbs and roll in the butter or oil. Lay out in the foil-lined pan, return to oven and bake uncovered about 15 minutes, or until golden brown. Serves two.

World's Best Oysters

    ¼   cup melted butter (or olive oil)
        Two splats Worcestershire sauce
    1   small splat prepared mustard
    3   tablespoons dry vermouth
        Oysters to serve two
        Coarse cracker crumbs

Moosh together the butter, Worcestershire, mustard and vermouth.

Bring a pan of water to a boil, drop in the oysters and when the water returns to a boil remove the oysters and rinse in cold water.

Dip the oysters in the sauce, roll in cracker crumbs and plunk on a cookie sheet topped with aluminum foil.

Bake in a 350-degree oven for 20 to 25 minutes or until the crumbs are golden brown. Add salt, pepper and lemon juice to taste.

If you don't have dry vermouth, you can use dry sherry. I used the Italian bread crumbs that come in a can, rather than cracker crumbs.

Some recipes suggest 10 ounces of medium oysters to serve two. Alice the Artists and I easily finished twice that much cooked in this fashion.

Oysters Florentine

    1 bunch spinach
    1 pint oysters
    ¼ cup Parmesan cheese
        Pinch of garlic powder
        Pinch of black pepper
    2 ounces ham (approximately)
    2 tablespoons butter
    1 tablespoon lemon juice
    ⅓ cup dry bread crumbs

Cook the spinach (you can substitute one package frozen). After it is cooked. drain the spinach and lay out in a lightly greased casserole. Top with the oysters and sprinkle with cheese, garlic powder and pepper.

Cut the ham into bits, saute in a small skillet until it begins to crisp up, and add to the casserole.

Combine melted butter and lemon juice and pour over everything.

Scatter the crumbs over the top and either dot with butter or spray with canola oil.

Bake the casserole 5 to 7 minutes in a 450-degree oven.

This will suffice for two eager eaters.

Casanova's Oysters

    ¼ cup butter or olive oil
    1 large onion, chopped
    1 teaspoon Italian herbs
    3 cloves garlic, chopped
    2 tablespoons chopped parsley
    ¼ teaspoon cayenne pepper
        Salt, pepper to taste
    1 quart oysters
    1 cup Italian style bread crumbs
    ½ cup Parmesan cheese

In a skillet melt the butter or heat the oil. Saute the onion (another love food) over medium heat until it begins to relax. Add all of the seasonings and the oysters with the oyster liquor (the liquid from the jar they came in).

Cook 1 minute then stir in crumbs.

Gloop everything into a buttered casserole, sprinkle with Parmesan and bake at 350 degrees for about 15 minutes. Serves four Norwegians or one amorous Italian.

Hay-Straw Stir Fry

    3 tablespoons olive oil
    1 pound bay scallops
    2 cloves garlic, minced
    2 small zucchini, sliced
    3 Italian tomatoes, chopped
    1 cup frozen peas
    1 teaspoon dried basil
    8 ounces hay and straw pasta
    1½ cups freshly grated romano or parmesan cheese

The original recipe, from the pioneer days in this area, called for real hay and straw.

Today when we talk about hay and straw pasta we're referring to mixed green and white spaghetti strands, which you can find in better markets. Or, buy packets of regular and spinach spaghetti and use four ounces of each in this recipe.

Heat a tablespoon of oil in a large skillet. Add the scallops and garlic and stir-fry two minutes. Remove to a warm bowl.

Add another tablespoon of oil to the skillet and saute the zucchini three minutes. Add tomatoes, basil and peas and cook one minute more.

Return scallop mixture to the pan. When reheated, pour contents of skillet over the cooked and drained pasta. Toss with the final tablespoon of oil, then scatter the grated cheese over the top. This will serve four.

Sauteed Scallop Spaghetti

    ½ pound pasta
    4 tablespoons olive oil
    ½ pound bay scallops
        salt, pepper
        flour
    1 clove garlic, minced
    3 tablespoons white wine
    ½ teaspoon oregano
    4 tablespoons pesto
    3 tablespoons warm water

Cook the pasta in boiling, salted water. Mix salt and pepper with flour and dredge scallops. Toss into pan with the hot oil, and stir-cook one minute. Add wine, garlic, oregano and cook another minute or two.

Plunk the pesto into a bowl. When pasta is cooked, spoon three tablespoons of the pot water in with the pesto. Drain the pasta and toss into a bowl. Add the scallops and pesto mixture and toss. Serves two to three.

Scallops Sicily

- 1 pound bay scallops
- ¾ pound penne or spiral pasta
- ½ teaspoon salt
- ½ teaspoon lemon pepper
- ¼ teaspoon garlic powder
- ¼ teaspoon onion powder
- ¼ teaspoon nutmeg
- 1 teaspoon chili powder
- ¼ teaspoon cayenne or less, to taste
- 2 tablespoons olive oil
- 1 cup chicken broth
- 1½ tablespoons cornstarch
- ½ cup no-fat or low-fat sour cream

In a bowl combine the salt, lemon pepper (or plain black pepper), garlic powder, onion powder, nutmeg, chili powder and cayenne. Toss the rinsed and drained scallops into a bowl, dump the spices on top and mix with your hands.

Cook the pasta in boiling salted water. Five minutes before it is cooked al dente, heat the oil in a skillet. Saute the scallops, tossing to cook on all sides, until they are barely done. Return the scallops to the bowl.

To the pan add the chicken broth and bring to a boil. Mix the cornstarch with a third of a cup of water and stir into the pan to thicken the sauce. Add the scallops and sour cream.

Drain the cooked pasta and dump into the skillet with the scallops and sauce. When mixed divide among four warm plates.

Dexterity Dinner

- ½ pound sea (large) scallops
- Milk
- Flour
- 1 tablespoon olive oil
- ¼ cup dry white wine
- ¼ cup chopped green onions
- Juice of one small lemon
- Lemon pepper

With the palm of your hand gently press the scallops to flatten slightly. Dip in milk then dredge in flour. Heat the oil in a skillet, add the scallops and cook briefly on both sides. When they are just done, remove to two ramekins, add the wine and green onions to the pan and simmer for a minute. Pour the sauce over the scallops, squeeze half a lemon over each ramekin and season to taste with lemon pepper.

Scallops to Flip Over

- 8 dried shiitake mushrooms
- 1 tablespoon soy sauce
- 1 tablespoon cornstarch
- 2 tablespoons dry white wine
- ½ pound bay scallops
- 3 tablespoon cooking oil
- 4 dried hot chilies
- 1 tablespoon minced fresh ginger
- 1 teaspoon minced garlic
- ½ cup sliced water chestnuts
- ½ cup sweet red pepper slices
- 2 tablespoons oriental oyster sauce
- 2 tablespoons minced green onion

Cover the mushrooms with warm water, let sit 30 minutes, then squeeze dry and slice. Rinse and pat dry the scallops. Cut the water chestnut slices in half. If you don't have oyster sauce you can use hoisin or teriyaki sauce. In a bowl moosh together the soy sauce, wine and cornstarch. Dump in the scallops and stir until coated.

Heat the oil in a skillet, toss in the dried chilies and remove after 30 seconds. Add the ginger and garlic and stir-cook a minute.

Lift the scallops out of the cornstarch muck, toss them into the pan and now you get to flip 'em. After six flips or 60 seconds, add the mushroom slices and red pepper. Flip again a few times, then stir in the water chestnuts and oyster sauce.

Moosh everything around for a minute, add the green onions, stir again, and serve in two ramekins, with cooked rice on the side.

Skillet Oysters

- 1 pint oysters
- ¼ cup butter or olive oil
- 1 cup fresh mushrooms, sliced
- 3 tablespoons cream
- ¼ teaspoon garlic powder
- Salt, pepper
- 3 eggs or egg substitute
- ¼ pound low-fat Swiss cheese, grated
- 1 tablespoon sherry
- Paprika to taste

Use a skillet with an ovenproof handle. (I warned you these recipes are almost too hot to handle.) Melt the butter in the pan and brown the mushrooms.

Add the cream, garlic powder and salt and pepper to taste. Reduce heat, plop in the grated cheese. Mix the sherry and oyster liquor with the lightly beaten eggs and add them to the pan, too. Distribute the oysters over the pan and sprinkle heavily with paprika.

Pour some hot water into a large oven pan and place on the rack of a 350-degree preheated oven. Transfer the skillet and its contents to the pan and bake – really, a kind of poach – for about 20 minutes. Turn on broiler briefly, if needed, to set the eggs.

This will serve two generously.

Shrimp-Scallop Cakes

   2 tablespoons butter or oil
   1 onion, minced
   ½ a green pepper, minced
   ½ a sweet red pepper, minced
   ½ pound small scallops
   ½ pound small shrimp
   1 egg, beaten (or egg substitute)
   ½ cup fresh bread crumbs
   ½ cup dry bread crumbs

Saute the onion in the butter or oil. If you have a food processor, use it to finely chop the scallops and shrimp. You can do this with a knife, but it will take a bit longer and you're still not going to get a big tip from me.

Mix the onion with the green and red peppers, the scallops, shrimp and fresh bread crumbs. Add salt and pepper to your taste. Then add the egg and moosh everything around.

Form the resultant muck into six patties. Coat with dry crumbs and saute in canola oil until golden on both sides. Serves three.

Feng Du Shrimp

   ½ pound medium prawns
   2 pounds of assorted veggies like broccoli, cabbage, fresh mushrooms, sliced carrots, pea pods and onions
   2 tablespoons Chinese oyster sauce
   2 cloves garlic, chopped
   1¼ cups chicken broth
   1 teaspoon black pepper
   2 tablespoons cooking oil
   ½ cup roasted cashews

Heat three-quarters of a cup of broth to a boil in a large pan. Add the vegetables for a minute, mooshing around with a spoon. Then dump the veggies and remaining sauce into a bowl.

In a skillet or wok, heat the cooking oil. Add the garlic and prawns and stir-cook for just 30 seconds. Add the veggies, oyster sauce and remaining chicken broth. Stir-cook until the shrimp are pink and the veggies have begun to relax. Add the black pepper and nuts, moosh around one more time, and serve to four guests with steamed rice on the side.

Shrimp Pie

   3 slices French bread, cubed
   1 cup milk
   2 cups cooked shrimp
   2 tablespoons melted butter
   3 eggs, well beaten (or egg substitute)
   ½ cup chopped green pepper
   ½ cup chopped celery
   1 teaspoon Worcestershire sauce
   2 tablespoons sherry
     Salt, pepper to taste
     Paprika

Soak bread in milk and mash with a fork. Add shrimp, butter, eggs, green pepper, celery, Worcestershire, sherry, salt and pepper. Turn into a buttered high-rim pie plate or small casserole and bake at 300 degrees for 20 to 30 minutes, or until almost set. Sprinkle with paprika, then shove under a broiler to brown top. Serves 3 to 4.

Fake Crab Cakes

   3 tablespoons cracker crumbs
   3 tablespoons mayonnaise
   1 teaspoon Dijon mustard
   1 tablespoon capers, drained
   ¼ cup minced parsley
   ¼ teaspoon salt
   ¼ teaspoon black pepper
     Pinch of cayenne pepper or to taste
   1 pound surimi (fake crab meat)
     Olive oil

Mix together the first eight ingredients. Fold in the fake crab meat and form into eight cakes. Saute on both sides in olive oil, until golden brown. Serve to four guests with wedges of lemon to squeeze over the top.

Scallops McMahon

   1 pound bay scallops
   1 tablespoon brown sugar, packed
   1 tablespoon soy sauce
   2 teaspoons cornstarch
     Quarter pound ham, cut in strips
   6 green onions in one-inch pieces
   1 can (8 oz.) sliced water chestnuts, drained
   4 ounces snow peas

Toss the scallops with the sugar, soy and cornstarch. Cover a skillet with a thin layer of cooking oil. Toss in the ham slivers and when they begin to sizzle add the scallops, onions and water chestnuts. Cook just until the scallops are white, then stir in the snow peas. Cook another minute or two then dish up onto four plates.

Baked Shrimp

    2 pounds large shrimp
    1 cube butter softened
    3 cloves garlic, mashed
    3 tablespoons sherry
    1 cup chopped fresh parsley leaves
    1 cup fine dry bread crumbs
    ¼ cup sliced almonds, slightly toasted

Preheat oven to 400 degrees.

Peel and devein the shrimp. Bring a pan of water to a boil, add salt and dump in the shrimp for a few seconds, just until they turn pink. Pour into strainer and cool with running water.

Cream together the butter, garlic, sherry, parsley and bread crumbs.

Scatter the shrimp in one layer over bottom of a greased oven dish. Spread the garlic butter gloop over the top. Top with a layer of almonds.

Bake for 15 minutes, basting once.

This should serve 6, along with French bread, a salad and potatoes that have been peeled, quartered, rubbed with oil, salt-and-peppered then shoved into the same oven about 45 minutes before you begin to cook the shrimp.

New Orleans Prawns

    ¾ pound prawns
    3 tablespoons olive oil
    1 teaspoon chili powder
    1 teaspoon freshly ground black pepper
    ⅛ teaspoon cayenne pepper
    1 medium clove garlic, minced
    2 teaspoons Worcestershire sauce
    2 tablespoons dry red wine
    ½ teaspoon salt or to taste

Shell the shrimp and lay out one layer deep in an oven dish.

In a small saucepan, heat all the other ingredients to a simmer. Then pour over the shrimp and put the dish into a 400-degree oven just until the shrimp are firm and pink, about eight minutes. Serve up on two plates with crusty bread for sopping up the juices.

Mazatlan Prawns

    2 pounds large prawns
    1 ounce olive oil
    2 ounces dry vermouth
    1 crushed clove garlic
    1 ounce butter
    Salt, pepper
    Juice of two lemons

Heat the olive oil in a large skillet. Toss in the shelled prawns and brown, tossing, for about half a minute. Lower heat and add the butter, garlic with salt and pepper to taste. Moosh around with a wooden spoon. Then add the lemon juice and vermouth and turn the heat up again for just one minute, stirring constantly.

Happy Clam Cioppino

    ¼ cup olive oil
    1 medium onion, chopped
    1 medium green pepper, seeded and chopped
    3 cloves garlic, minced or smashed
    1 14-ounce can chopped tomatoes
    1 10-ounce can tomato puree
    1½ cups dry red wine
    2 teaspoons dried oregano
    1 teaspoon dried basil
    1 teaspoon salt (or to taste)
    ¼ teaspoon pepper
    1 pound snapper or cod fillets
    1 pound medium prawns
    40 steamer clams

The reason I use 40 clams is because that's the limit for one digger where I live.

But first shell the prawns and cover the shells with two cups of boiling water.

Then saute the onions and green pepper in the olive oil in a large pot.

When the onion begins to relax, add the garlic and cook another minute. Then add the tomatoes, tomato puree, the prawn-shell water (discarding the shells), the red wine, oregano, basil, salt and pepper. Simmer for about 12 minutes.

Cut the fish into 1 ½-inch chunks and add to the pot. Toss in the shelled prawns, too.

After two minutes add the clams and cover the pot.

When all the clams open you are ready to serve this up for four to six guests with French bread and a tossed salad.

If you like a spicier cioppino, toss some cayenne pepper or dried red pepper flakes into the pot when you are adding the other seasonings. Or, considering that some guests may not like it as hot as you do, keep a jar of Chinese hot chili sauce with garlic on the table and let people add as much to their bowls as they desire.

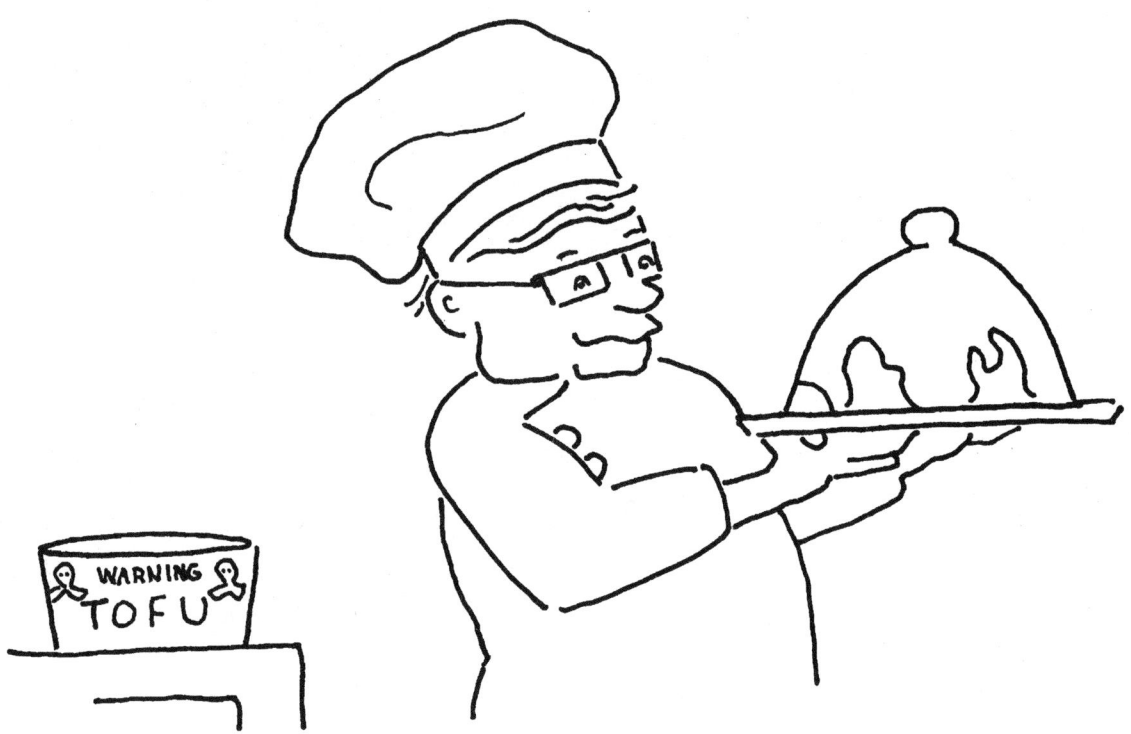

DESSERTS

Presumably food writers receive similar correspondence from their readers.

If so, I wish somebody would reveal their stock answer to the question:

"Why don't you ever run any good recipes for tofu?"

The logical answer, which I only mutter under my breath, is that there are no good recipes for tofu.

OK, I concede tofu is a complete protein, with lots of B vitamins, iron and phosphorus. It is free of saturated fat and cholesterol, low in sodium. So why do I have this prejudice against it?

Probably because it tastes like iron and phosphorus, is free of saturated fat and is dreadfully low in sodium.

Legend has it that tofu was "discovered" about 2,000 years ago when some sea salt with coagulating properties was accidentally spilled into a vat of heated soybean milk and began to form curds.

I'd hate to tell you all the accidents that have occurred in my kitchen. But I have never written a letter to Julia Child prefaced, "Why don't you ever run any good recipes for a sardine and anchovy pate that has sort of turned black but glows in the dark after sitting hidden behind a mango chutney jar in my refrigerator for the last nine months?"

I've tried tofu burgers (iron and phosphorus between a bun with a slice of pickle). I've tried Chinese tofu stir-fry concoctions (vitamin B smashed into a custard and sauteed in oyster sauce).

Believe me, you don't want my recipe.

Then somebody recommended that I use tofu as a substitute ingredient in one of my favorite dessert recipes. I tried it in this one and (shazam!) it was not only edible, it was sensational. The recipe is on the next page.

Crisp With Tofu Cream

- 6 large red-skinned apples
- 1 tablespoon lemon juice
- ½ cup raisins
- ½ cup chopped walnuts
- 1 cup sugar
- 1 teaspoon ground cinnamon
- ½ teaspoon ground nutmeg
- ¾ cup flour
- 1/3 cup butter
- ¾ cup tofu
- 1 cup skim milk

Peel, core and thickly slice the apples to make eight cups. In a large bowl, mix together the apple slices, lemon juice, raisins, nuts, half cup of the sugar and the cinnamon and nutmeg.

When mixed, dump into a 9-inch-square pan. Combine the remaining half-cup sugar with the flour. Cut in the butter until you have a crumbly mixture, then scatter over the top of the apple mixture.

Bake uncovered in a 400-degree oven for 45 minutes and serve warm topped with tofu cream. (In a blender or processor plunk ¾ cup tofu and one cup skim milk. Process for a full minute.)

Christmas Cake

- 1 cup sifted cake flour
- 1/3 cup unsweetened cocoa
- 1 teaspoon baking soda
- 1 teaspoon baking powder
- Whites of six large eggs
- 1 1/3 cups firmly packed brown sugar
- 1 cup plain, nonfat yogurt
- 1 teaspoon vanilla
- Powdered sugar

As you can see, this is a low-fat formula for a cake as light as an angel's kiss.

Mix together the flour, cocoa, baking soda and baking powder. In a large bowl, beat the egg whites with the brown sugar, yogurt and vanilla until smooth. Add flour mixture and stir just until everything is moistened.

Spray a 9-inch-square baking pan with oil, and dust lightly with flour.

Pour the cake sludge into the pan. Bake in a preheated 350-degree oven until done, usually 30 to 40 minutes. Let cake cool 15 minutes, then invert on a serving plate.

Sift the powdered sugar over the top of the cake. Using a paper cutout, Alice creates a snowflake pattern with the powdered sugar.

You can serve the cake warm or cold.

Earth-Friendly Apple Crisp

- 4 tart apples
- 1 teaspoon cinnamon
- 1 teaspoon salt
- ¼ cup water
- 1/3 cup flour
- 1/3 cup oatmeal
- 1 cup brown sugar
- ¼ cup butter or substitute

Core the apples, slice and lay out in a buttered 9-by-9-inch oven dish. Mix together the cinnamon, salt and water. Sprinkle this mess over the apples.

Combine in a bowl the flour, oatmeal, sugar and butter. (Or use canola oil and Butter Buds.) Rub together with your fingers then spread over the apples. Shove the dish into a 350-degree oven for 40 minutes.

Cranberry Cake

- 2¼ cups sifted flour
- 1 cup sugar
- ¼ teaspoon salt
- 1 teaspoon baking powder
- 1 teaspoon baking soda
- 1 cup chopped walnuts
- 1 cup dates, diced
- 1 cup fresh, whole cranberries
- Grated rind of two oranges
- 2 eggs, beaten (or egg substitute)
- 1 cup buttermilk
- ¾ cup canola oil
- 1 cup orange juice
- 1 cup sugar
- Vanilla ice cream

Sift together into a bowl the flour, sugar, salt, baking powder and baking soda. Stir in the nuts, dates, cranberries and orange rind.

Moosh together in another bowl the eggs, buttermilk and canola oil. Dump this mess into the bowl with the dry ingredients. Stir together until blended while humming the alto part of a 15th-century composition for massed choir and electric guitar.

Pour into a well-buttered 10-inch tube pan and bake in a 350-degree oven for an hour. Remove from the oven, let cool in the pan until lukewarm. Then remove to a rack which has been placed over a bowl.

Moosh together the orange juice and sugar. Pour over the cake.

Serve with non-fat vanilla yogurt. If you want to keep the cake for a day or two, cover with foil and refrigerate.

Floating Islands

- 2 tablespoons gelatin
- 1½ cup whipping cream
- ½ cup sugar
- ¼ cup plain yogurt
- ¾ cup sour cream
- ½ teaspoon vanilla
- 2 tablespoons orange liquor

In a saucepan soften the gelatin in one tablespoon of cold water. Then add the cream and sugar. Warm over medium heat, stirring, until gelatin has dissolved. Do not boil. Remove from heat and dump the ingredients into a bowl.

Let cool 30 minutes, stirring twice. Stir in the yogurt, sour cream, vanilla and orange liquor. I used L'Orange Napoleon liquor, but you can use Grand Marnier or a similar product.

Divide this muck between six glass bowls, cover with plastic wrap and refrigerate for at least an hour.

For the sauce:

- 3 10-ounce packages of frozen raspberries
- 2 tablespoons Framboise, kirsch or other berry liquor
- Sprigs of mint

Puree the thawed berries with the berry liquor. If you have access to fresh raspberries and want to use them instead, add one tablespoon of sugar.

To serve the desserts, spread six plates with lakes of raspberry sauce. Unmold the floating islands and plunk each in the center of the sauce.

Garnish with fresh sprigs of mint.

Santa Fe Strawberry Pie

- 6 cups fresh strawberries
- ¾ cup sugar
- 3 tablespoons cornstarch
- 1 teaspoon grated orange peel
- 6 tablespoons water
- 2 tablespoons thawed orange juice concentrate
- Baked, 9-inch pie crust

Hull the washed fruit. Combine the sugar, cornstarch and orange peel in a pan.

In a blender, puree 2 cups strawberries with the 6 tablespoons of water. Pour this sludge into the pan with the sugar mixture. Cook to a full boil, then stir in the orange concentrate.

Arrange the remaining whole berries in the cooked crust. Evenly spoon the glaze over the top. Refrigerate the pie, covered, for at least 1 hour.

Filibuster Bars

- ½ cup butter
- ½ cup white sugar
- Grated rind of one lemon
- 1½ cups flour
- 2 large eggs (or egg substitute)
- 1 cup firmly packed brown sugar
- ¼ teaspoon baking powder
- 1 cup chopped walnuts

Cream the butter, the white sugar and half the lemon rind. Gradually stir in 1¼ cups of flour. Press evenly over the bottom of a 13-by-9-inch baking pan. Bake in a preheated 350-degree oven about 15 minutes, or until golden.

Meanwhile, beat eggs slightly. Add brown sugar, remaining lemon rind, remaining flour and the baking powder. Stir over low heat until smooth. Stir in walnuts. Spread mixture over the hot baked crust and bake for 20 minutes in a 350-degree oven.

Place on wire rack to cool slightly. Spread with glaze while still warm.

Glaze:

- 1 cup powdered sugar
- 1 tablespoon softened butter
- 2 tablespoons lemon juice

Blend together until smooth. Then spread as directed above. Cool completely, then cut the dessert into bars. You should have about 36.

Okanogan Peach Pie

- 1 quart sliced peaches
- 3 tablespoons cornstarch
- 1/3 cup water
- 1 tablespoon lemon juice
- Pinch of salt
- 1 cup sugar
- 1 9-inch, deep dish pie crust

Bake your favorite pie crust in the tin and let cool.

You'll need five to six peaches and it's OK if some of them seem overly ripe. Peel and slice, then dump half the peaches (the ripest ones) into a blender or food processor. Add the cornstarch, mixed with water, and lean on the button until you have a peach puree. Dump into a microwaveable dish and stir in the lemon juice, salt and sugar.

Place the puree mixture in a microwave oven and cook 6 minutes on high, removing every minute or so to stir the mixture with a wooden spoon. When the puree has cooked and thickened, remove from the oven and let cool about 15 minutes.

Arrange the rest of the peach slices in the cooked pie crust. Pour the puree mixture over the top and refrigerate the pie until set. You can serve as is, or top with a bit of low-fat whipped cream or soft ice cream.

Chili Powder Pie

- 4 large pie apples
- ¾ cup sugar
- 2 tablespoons butter or canola oil
- 1 teaspoon ground cinnamon
- ½ teaspoon ground nutmeg
- 2 teaspoons chili powder
- 1 cup water
- ¼ teaspoon salt
- Double crust for 9-inch pie plate

Peel the apples, core and slice. Plunk them into a pot with the sugar, butter, spices, salt and water. Simmer about 25 minutes or until slices are tender and the liquid has reduced.

Dump this mess into an uncooked crust in a 9-inch pie pan. Top with the second crust, moisten edges and pinch together. Cut four vents into the top crust and shove the pie into a preheated 375-degree oven for 30 to 40 minutes.

Serve warm with vanilla ice cream.

I have used frozen crusts to make this pie and it still won raves from chili-heads, southpaw pitchers and other peculiar people.

Easy Biscotti

- 1¾ cups flour
- 2 teaspoons baking powder
- ¾ cup slivered almonds
- 2 eggs or egg substitute
- ¾ cup sugar
- ⅓ cup butter, softened
- 2 teaspoons vanilla
- 1 teaspoon almond extract
- 2 teaspoons grated orange peel
- 1 egg white, lightly beaten

In a large mixing bowl, combine the flour, baking powder and almonds. In another smaller bowl mix together the eggs, sugar, butter, vanilla, almond extract and orange peel. Whisk to incorporate, then stir into the flour mixture.

When thoroughly mixed, moosh the sticky dough up in your hands and dump it on a floured board. Roll and knead briefly, sprinkling with a bit of flour if needed, just until it is no longer sticky.

Cut the dough in half and form into two 12-inch logs. Place on a greased baking sheet and brush the exposed surfaces with the egg white. Bake 20 minutes in a preheated, 350-degree oven.

Remove from oven, let cool 6 minutes on a rack, then slice the loaves diagonally into ¾-inch pieces. Return them to the baking pan, standing upright.

Return pan to the 350-degree oven for another 20-25 minutes. Cool on rack and store in airtight container.

Lime Pie

- 1 can (13 ounces) condensed milk
- 4 eggs, separated
- ½ cup lime juice
- 1 frozen 9-inch pie crust
- 6 tablespoons sugar
- ½ teaspoon cream of tartar

Moosh together the condensed milk, egg yolks and lime juice. (Some of the better markets in Seattle sell genuine Key lime juice.) Fold in one egg white, which has been beaten stiff. Pour this sludge into the crust.

Beat the remaining 3 egg whites and gradually add the sugar and cream of tartar. Spread over the top of the pie and shove into a preheated 350-degree oven until egg whites are golden brown, about 20 minutes.

Dmitri's Dessert

- 6 firm pears
- 6 tablespoons butter, chilled
- ½ cup flour
- ⅓ cup firmly packed brown sugar
- Grated zest of one lemon
- ½ teaspoon ground cinnamon
- ¼ teaspoon freshly ground nutmeg
- ¼ teaspoon ground allspice
- ½ cup lightly toasted pecans
- 3 tablespoons brandy, rum or bourbon

Peel, halve and core the pears, then cut into ¼-inch slices. Grease a 9-by-13-inch oven dish and layer the pears over the bottom.

Dump the butter, flour, sugar, lemon zest and spices into a processor and lean on the button until you have coarse crumbs. Stir in the pecans, and pour this mess over the pears. Drizzle with booze and shove the dish into a 350-degree oven for 15 minutes. Serve warm with coffee latte yogurt or ice cream.

That's a classic dessert and a departure from the low-fat theme. But each serving will still include only one tablespoon of butter.

Maple Bars

The Bars:

    2 eggs or egg substitute
    1 cup sugar
    ⅔ cup canola oil
    1 cup flour
    ½ teaspoon salt
    ½ teaspoon baking powder
    ½ teaspoon nutmeg
    ½ teaspoon cinnamon
    ¼ teaspoon allspice
    2 cups walnuts, chopped
    1 cup raisins
    2 teaspoons maple flavoring

    Beat together the eggs, sugar and oil.
    Sift the flour, salt and baking powder together. Mix in the nutmeg, cinnamon and allspice. Dump these dry ingredients into the egg-sugar muck.
    Stir in the walnuts, raisins and maple flavoring. (If you dislike raisins, leave 'em out.)
    Spread the batter into a greased, 9-by-13-inch oven dish or pan. Bake in oven, preheated to 350 degrees, for 25 to 30 minutes, or until the oven alarm chases the cat up the chimney.
    When done, remove from oven and let cool. Then pour this over the top:

The Frosting:

    6 tablespoons milk
    6 tablespoons brown sugar, packed
    2 tablespoons butter
    ⅛ teaspoon salt
    ¼ teaspoon maple flavoring
    2 cups powdered sugar

    Combine in a pan the milk and brown sugar. Bring to a bare boil, stirring.
    Plunk the butter into a bowl and top with the hot sugar mixture. Beat until incorporated, then add the salt and maple flavoring. Gradually add the powdered sugar until this mess looks and acts like frosting. If it is too thick add a little milk.
    After frosting, cut this toothsome snack into bars (you should have between 18 and 24.)

Peanut Butter Cookies

    1 cup crunchy peanut butter
    ½ cup canola oil
    ¼ teaspoon salt
    ¾ cup sugar
    ¾ cup brown sugar
    2 well-beaten eggs (or egg substitute)
    1 tablespoon milk
    1 cup sifted flour
    ¼ teaspoon baking soda
    ¼ teaspoon ginger

    In the large bowl of an electric mixer combine the peanut butter, oil and salt. (I used Jiff Extra Crunchy peanut butter.) Blend well, then add the two sugars, the eggs and milk.
    Into a separate bowl, sift together the flour, soda and ginger. Gradually stir this into the peanut butter gloop.
    Chill the mixture until you can form into small balls. Place them on an ungreased cookie sheet, press top with a fork and bake for 15 to 20 minutes in a 325-degree oven. Cool the cookies on a wire rack.

Refudgerators

    ½ cup canola oil
    2½ ounces unsweetened baking chocolate
    ¼ cup granulated sugar
    2 cups graham cracker crumbs
    1 cup coconut
    ½ cup chopped nuts
    2 teaspoons vanilla extract
    1 egg, beaten
    ¼ cup butter
    2 cups powdered sugar
    1 tablespoon milk

    In large saucepan, heat oil and 1 ounce chocolate. Stir in the granulated sugar, graham cracker crumbs, coconut, nuts, one teaspoon vanilla and the egg. Mix well and press into a 9-by-11-inch dish or pan and chill while you prepare the next layer.
    Cream the ¼ cup butter with powdered sugar, 1 teaspoon vanilla and the milk. Spread smoothly over the chilled bottom layer.
    Melt the remaining 1½ ounces of chocolate, cool slightly and dribble over the top layer. Cool in refrigerator until firm, then cut into squares.

Nitty Gritty Pudding

1 14-ounce can Eagle brand condensed milk
1½ cups cold water
1 package (4 serving size) instant vanilla pudding mix
2 cups whipping cream, whipped (or low-fat substitute)
36 vanilla wafers
3 medium bananas, sliced and dipped in lemon juice

In large bowl mix together sweetened condensed milk and water. Add pudding mix and beat well. Chill 5 minutes. Whip cream (I used chilled evaporated milk) and fold into the pudding. Spoon 1 cup of this mess into a glass serving bowl. Top with 1/3 each of wafers, bananas and pudding. Repeat layers twice ending with pudding. Cover and chill.

Makes 8-10 servings and it's best if you finish it by the second day.

Gingerbread for John

1 can (20 ounces) sliced apples
1 teaspoon cinnamon
1 teaspoon lemon juice
½ teaspoon grated lemon peel
1¼ cups flour
1 teaspoon ginger
½ teaspoon cinnamon
¼ teaspoon salt
¼ teaspoon ground cloves
¼ cup butter
½ cup sugar
1 egg
½ cup molasses
½ teaspoon baking soda
½ cup boiling water
Whipped cream

You can usually find the sliced apples in the baking section of the supermarket.

Mix the apples with the cinnamon, lemon juice and peel. Spread it into a greased 9-by-9-inch baking pan.

Sift next five ingredients into a bowl.

In a larger bowl cream the butter with the sugar. Mix in the egg and molasses and beat until smooth.

Dissolve the baking soda in the boiling water. Alternately add the flour mixture and hot water to the molasses mixture, beating. Pour this mess over the apples and shove the pan into a preheated 350-degree oven. Bake for 45 minutes or until a toothpick comes out clean when stuck in the middle.

Serve warm in squares with whipped cream.

Cottage Pudding

1¾ cups sifted flour
2 teaspoons baking powder
½ teaspoon salt
¼ cup soft butter
¾ cup sugar
1 large egg
¾ cup milk
1 teaspoon vanilla

Sift together the flour, baking powder and salt. Add the other ingredients and beat until smooth. Pour into a 9-inch-square pan that has been both greased and sprinkled with flour.

Bake in a 350-degree oven for 30 minutes or until done. Serve with:

Welsh Sauce:

1 cup sugar
2 tablespoons cornstarch
2 cups boiling water
2 tablespoons butter
2 teaspoons vanilla
½ teaspoon nutmeg

Mix the sugar and cornstarch together in a saucepan. Gradually stir in the hot water. Boil one minute, stirring. Then stir in the butter, vanilla and nutmeg.

Dish up the cottage pudding in squares, pour sauce over the top and if there is a better dish than this then Shawn Kemp is a Huggy Bear.

Monday's Sundaes

1 10-ounce carton frozen raspberries
2 tablespoons butter
2 tablespoons rum
1 pint low-fat vanilla ice cream or frozen yogurt
1 pint strawberries, halved
Whipping cream

Puree the thawed raspberries with their syrup in a blender. Strain into a saucepan to remove seeds and simmer 3 minutes. Add the butter and rum and cool to room temperature.

Place a scoop of ice cream in each of four dishes, arrange the strawberries around each scoop and top with the raspberry sauce and whipped cream.

Gifts for Friends

To order additional copies of Gluttony Without Guilt send $14.95 per book (plus $2.25 tax and shipping) to:
P-I Public Affairs Department, Box 1909, Seattle, WA 98111-1909.

INDEX

A

Airline Loaves 9
All-Day Cassoulet 34
Another Veggie-Mac 25
Ancient Healing Stir Fry 59
Antipasto Spread 40
Apple Crisp 74
Apricot Chicken 48
Aquatic Pork Chops 64
Artichoke Chicken 47
Artichoke Salad 18
Artichokes 25
Asparachick 31

B

Baked Clams 40
Baked Shrimp 72
Balsamic Salmon 65
Banana Pudding 78
Beanareeno 35
Beef Stir-Fry 59
Bean Dip 39
Beans 34, 35
Bed Time Spread 39
Beefy Potato Roast 23
Bird Feeder Muffins 8
Biscotti 76
Black Beans and Rice 34
Boiled Bird Feast 52
Bread 8, 9
Broccoli 22

C

Cabbage 26
Cable Car Rice 35
Cadillac Chicken 46
Calcutta Chicken 51
California Carrots 24
California Liver 60
Calamari 63, 65
Capt. Cook's Rice 35
Capt. Midnight Muffins 8
Capt. Rafferty's Loaf 59
Carolina Collards 22
Carrots 24
Casanova's Oysters 69
Cassoulet 34
Cauliflower 23, 24
Cauliflower Curry 23
Cauliflower Ear 24
Cedar St. Corn Cakes 10
Charlie's Salad 19
Cheese Potatoes 23
Chickadee Salad 18
Chicken Dishes 46-54
Chicken and Mushrooms 48
Chicken Salad 18
Chicken Vesuvio 48
Chili Chicken Soup 12
Chili 14-15
Chili Powder Pie 76
China Burgers 52
Christmas Cake 74
Christmas Eve Casserole 28
Cioppino 72
Clam Chowder 16
Clams, Baked 40
Clucker Snacks 39
Collards 22, 26
Company Chicken Salad 18
Computer Pork Roast 56
Corn Cakes 10
Corn Soup 16
Cottage Pudding 78
Coyote Salad 18
Crackers 39
Cranberry Cake 74
Crisp With Tofu Cream 74
Cross-Country Casserole 32
Curried Lentil Soup 15

D

Dexterity Dinner 70
Dijon Sole 66
Dmitri's Dessert 76
Dinner for Dummies 54
Drumsticks, Chicken 40
Drumstick Dinner, Turkey 46
Duffer's Gravy 54

E

Easy Biscotti 76
Earth Friendly Apple Crisp 74
Eat-Your Broccoli 22
Edmonds Toast 9
Emerald City Manicotti 43
Enchiladas 30

F

Fake Crab Cakes 71
Far East Chicken 50
Far Out Fish 62
Feng Du Shrimp 71
Father's Day Feast 53
Filibuster Bars 75
Filibuster Chili 15
Flank Steak 57-60
Floating Islands 75
Foiled Trout 63
Frankly Flank 57
French Fish 66
French Toast 9
Fried Rice 36

G

Garbure 15
Gazpacho Guadalahara 20
Georgian Stew 57
Ginger Beef 60
Ginger Broccoli 22

Ginger Fried Rice 36
Gingerbread for John 78
Glacier Bay Beef 56
Gold Medal Munchies 39
Golf Balls 54
Gopher's Game Hens 50
Graham Bread 9
Great Western Muffins 8
Greek Salad 19
Green Bean Casserole 24
Green Olive Pesto 43
Green Onion Fillets 62
Greens 26
Ground Turkey Spaghetti Sauce 51

H

Halibut 62, 65
Ham-Noodle Casserole 32
Happy Clam Cioppino 72
Happy Holiday Lasagne 42
Hash Brown Quiche 10
Hawaiian Chicken 49
Hawaiian Cornbread 9
Hawaiian Halibut 65
Hay-Straw Stir Fry 69
Herb Crackers 39
Herbed Mussels 68
Holiday Herb Crackers 39
Hoover Hazelnut Rice 36
Homerun Noodles 44
Hook, Line, Sinker 62
Hornby Island Halibut 62
Hungarian Cabbage 26

I

Icicle Creek Soup 12

J

Java Ginger Beef 60
Jimica Salad 20
Jungle Dip 38

K

Kauai Chicken 47

L

Last Best Steak 57
Lasagne 42
Leavenworth Chicken 51
Lemon Chicken Caper 46
Like Chocolate for Chicken 49
Lime Pie 76
Limustard Salmon 65
Liver 59, 60
Liver Trattoria 59
Low Budget Fish Stew 64
Lucky's Tomato Soup 14

M

Macaroni and Cheese 31
Macaroni Veggies 25
Maestro's Manicotti 42
Manicotti 42, 43
Maple Bars 77
Mazatlan Prawns 72
McPasta 44
Meat Ball Soup 12
Meat Balls 58
Meat Loaf 59
Mexican Beans 35
Mexican Shrimp Salad 20
Mint Pesto for Salmon 63
Mole Chicken 53
Monday's Sundaes 78
Muffins 8
Mulligaturkey Soup 16
Mussels 68
Multi-Vitamin Broccoli 22
Mustard Pea Soup 13
Myrtle's Calamari 63

N

Navajo Stew 58
Near East Feast 30
New Age Sausage Snack 38
New Orleans Prawns 72
Nitty Gritty Pudding 78
No-Neurosis Enchiladas 30
Noodles 44
Normandy Mussels 68
Norma's Chicken 49

O

Okanogan Peach Pie 75
Olympia Wild Rice 36
Olympic Drumroll Drumsticks 40
One Dish Dinner 54
Onion-Flavored Flank 58
Onion Soup 12
Open-Faced Option 49
Oven Oysters 68
Oysters 68-70
Oysters Florentine 69
Oyster Stew 16

P

Paella 29
Panhandle Pork Chops 56
Pea and Barley Bowl 15
Peach Pie 75
Peanut Butter Cookies 77
Peanut Pasta 44
Pear Crisp 76
Pecos Parmesan Steak 57
Pender St. Noodles 44
Picnic Potato Salad 18
Pipeline Beans 35
Pollo Extra-Olive 50
Pork Chops 56
Pork Loin 56
Pork Vindaloo 58
Portuguese Bean Soup 13
Portuguese Chicken 47
Potatoes 23
Potato Cakes 10
Potato Salad 18
Potato-Pea Salad 19
Puget Potato Cakes 10
Prawn Appetizer 40
Puffin Pasta 43
Pumpkin Spread 9
Punjabi Soup 14

Q

Quiche 10
Quick Veggie Soup 13

R

Red and Green Beans 24
Refudgerators 77
Rice 35, 36
Rice-Cabbage Salad 20
Roasted Pork Loin 56
Route 101 Zucchini Bread 8

S

Safari Stir-Fry 22
Sage-Garlic Chicken 51
Salads, 18-20
Salmon 63-65
Salmon Cakes 64
Salmon Loaf 64
Salmon Spuds 64
Salpicon 38
Salsa 28
Santa Fe Strawberry Pie 75
Sausage Snack 38
Sauteed Scallop Spaghetti 69
Scallops 69-71
Scallops to Flip Over 70
Scallops McMahon 71
Scallops Sicily 70
Scandi Meatballs 58
Seacombe Salmon 63
Seafood Italian 29
Sexy Spread 39
Shiver My Liver 59
Shrimp 71-72
Shrimp Pie 71

Shrimp Salad 20
Shrimp-Scallop Cakes 71
Skater's Thighs 48
Skillet Oysters 70
Sloppy Toms 52
Smoked Chicken 53
Snappy Snapper 65
Sole 66
Solidarity Squid 65
Soup, 12-16
Southern Greens 26
Spaghetti Sauce 51
Special Salsa 28
Stiragus 25
Strawberry Pie 75
Stir Fry 59
Sue Ellen's Salmon Loaf 64
Sweetbreads for Sweethearts 60
Sweet Corn Soup 16
Swiss and Spinach 29

T

Tapenade Parisian 40
Ten Minute Turkey Dinner 50
Teriyaki Sauce 38
Three-B Casserole 36
Tofu Cream 74
Trout 63
Tuna Casseroles 28
Tuna Salad 19
Turkey Balls 38
Turkey, boiled 52

Turkey Casseroles 28, 32
Turkey Drumstick Dinner 46
Turkey Meat Loaf 54
Turkey Soup 16
Turkey Stuffing 52
Twice-Cooked Spuds 23
Two Thousand Year Soup 14

U

Unstuffed Stuffing 52

V

Van Gogh's Paella 29
Vegetable Soup 13

W

Walnut Sauce 47
Wayne's Spinach 26
Welsh Soup 13
Wild Bill's Beans 34
Wild Turkey Casserole 28
World's Best Oysters 68

Y

Yakima Valley Chili 14

Z

Zucchini Parmesan 24

 **NOTES**

 # NOTES

 **NOTES**

 # NOTES